ASTHMA BEGINS AT HOME

HELP YOURSELF TO A HEALTHIER FUTURE

ROSIE GORDON

EMERALD PUBLISHING
www.straightforwardco.co.uk

Emerald Publishing Ltd
Brighton
East Sussex
BN2 4EG

British Library Cataloguing in Publication Data. A catalogue record
of this book is available from the British Library.

ISBN 1847160263
ISBN 13: 9781847160 26 3
Printed by Biddles Ltd Kings Lynn Norfolk

Cartoons by Waldorf, info@cambridge-associates.co.uk

ASTHMA BEGINS AT HOME

TABLE OF CONTENTS

Chapter Four

. . . .

ASTHMA BEGINS AT HOME
PREFACE

Millions of people are sick with allergic asthma, despite the millions of pounds that are ploughed into researching it each year. Why?

I have written this in order to get Nell Nockles' research through to the general public. It's our belief that we could and should be saving lives now, through simple changes in the home. But, in a world dominated by pharmaceutical companies, it's not surprising that 'Angry from Surrey' isn't getting much attention.

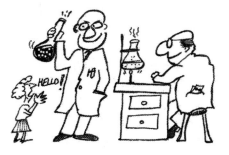

If Nell hadn't stumbled on a discovery about her bedroom and the damage it was doing to her health, I am not sure she'd still be here. It's our duty to pass on all the subsequent research she has done to you, so that you can improve your health and, most importantly, that of your children. We have seen great health improvements in children and family life following Nell's simple methods. Remember, the information in this book is based upon the independent research of someone who has experienced serious asthma. Much of the information is from other studies, government funded or independent, that we have dug up.

Many of you will already know that you are allergic to the house dust mite and other things, and have some idea about how to clean up your environment. This book is designed to enlighten you a little further; to help you **really** understand asthma and the damage it does. It is also designed to help you educate your children about making healthier life choices. I know you want to learn this stuff – we get hundreds of enquiries from allergy sufferers and worried parents through our website. I hope this book inspires you to do more research, taking control of your own healthy, active life.

I'm not pretending to be a doctor, nurse or scientist. These are the people whom you should always consult for medical advice. Equally, I am not a 'quack'. I'm simply questioning the cynicism that many people have towards alternative approaches (anything not endorsed by pharmaceutical companies, if we're being cynical). Why NOT do your own research and keep an open mind?

In the UK, our government is now keen to focus on educating people about controlling health problems by taking more responsibility for their lifestyle. This is because it has realised that the spending on medication is running away with us. In a sense, we need to get 'back to basics' and take more responsibility for preventing health problems ourselves.

Maybe, if we can break the cycle of ill health - which comes about through lack of education, rubbishy chemical food, stuffy, humid homes and our modern sedentary lifestyle - future generations will see a decline in asthma and allergy levels. The world will be richer on every level. We need to stop depending on drugs and help ourselves a little.

Rosie Gordon

rosie@nockles.com

www.housedustmite.org

8

The Tale of The
Angry Asthmatic

How many people do you know that have given up their social life, wealth, future comfort and security, and every waking hour, to the cause of fighting for information to be given to the public?

Back in 1997, Nell Nockles was formally diagnosed with asthma. She had suffered acute chronic coughing all her life but the actual diagnosis of asthma wasn't made until she was in her fifties. As a child, Nell's coughing often disrupted her family life and schooling. She was always tired, due to broken nights or constant bouts of 'colds'. She'd been on medication all her life, which was a norm in the USA. As a married woman (now in the UK), Nell's husband and children could tell where she was by listening for her relentless cough, which just got worse as she got older. Her family lived in constant fear of her death. Lack of sleep because of coughing, combined with the loss of taste or smell, resulted in constant trips to the doctor to try something new. By the time the doctor referred Nell to a specialist consultant to have her sinuses scraped, she was resigned to a very poor quality of life and was willing to go through an extremely painful operation just to have some sort of 'normal' life.

Around the same time, a family friend and doctor in respiratory medicine talked to Nell about her asthma. He casually mentioned to her that she should avoid house dust mites. He said no more about it, but Nell's interest was aroused. She looked up house dust mites at the library and found one paperback book, 'House Dust Mites - How they affect asthma, eczema and other allergies', by Des Whitrow. After reading the book, Nell realised that these mites were probably thriving in her bedroom and may even be a cause of her coughing.

She was doubtful, but desperate and dreading the sinus operation, Nell thought she might as well give this theory a shot. In order to change her environment, she moved into the study and slept on an inflatable mattress on the desk, which she knew would deny mites a breeding ground. The room had no carpet, and plenty of ventilation. Within two to three weeks, Nell's chronic coughing stopped. This had not happened for years. She found she could taste and smell food again. The relief was indescribable. She cancelled her sinus operation and began to think about the implications of this change in her health and quality of life.

It was obvious to Nell that this little experiment was a potential answer to improving the health of thousands of people. She was beginning to realise that asthmatics might have some control over their symptoms. When Nell made contact with the author Des Whitrow and went to visit her at her home in Nottingham, Des told her that the dust mite book had not been well received. She said that the issue of house dust mites in asthma did not seem to have been taken very seriously by doctors.

Nell knew first hand that this 'issue' should be taken seriously. She was becoming increasingly angry that she had only stumbled across her new knowledge by chance. Why hadn't she been given advice about dust mites years ago? She had lived with breathing troubles and illness for over fifty years without knowing about these creatures.

At the British Library, Nell's life as a scientific researcher took off. The brilliant staff there taught her how to research and reference properly, and her search threw up a huge amount of valuable information. She spent so much time researching there that she was asked to pose for a photograph for the Library's 2000/2001 annual report!

As Nell's research progressed, her anger, instead of abating, grew. There was so much 'buried' information, dating back for years, about house dust mites and the effect they had on allergic people. She discovered that 85 per cent of asthmatics were allergic to house dust mites – so why wasn't the information out in the public eye? Why had she, and millions like her, been suffering debilitating symptoms that they could have done something about? Nell decided that it would be her personal mission to translate the medical notes she was reading into a simple, practical form for the public.

Nell went on to produce a special bed and educational materials for asthmatic children. She took part in a clinical study (see Chapter Three), launched an information website and now continues to campaign for an open line of communication between scientists and the general public. To summarise, she is fighting for your right to choose a healthier future, and your right to understand this disease.

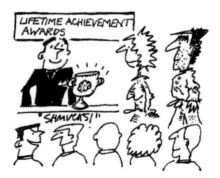

Because asthma is so common these days, people tend to assume that there is nothing they can (or should) do about it. At the moment, most asthmatics are relying on drugs to get through life. But their health is not improving, and the modern asthma epidemic is spreading. Can this really be the right approach?

We believe that the day you realise that you can do something to help yourself is the day you start to get better.

A Matter of Facts

If you still need convincing that there is something inefficient about the way the western world is dealing with asthma, read on:

300 million people around the world are asthmatic and the number is growing by 50 per cent every decade.
(World Health Organisation)

Asthma is responsible for some 180,000 deaths a year.
(BBC)

There are an estimated 1,500 to 3,000 new cases of occupational asthma each year. This rises to 7,000 cases a year if you include asthma made worse by work (work-related asthma).
(Health and Safety Executive)

The economic costs of treating asthma and days of work lost through illness are estimated to exceed those for tuberculosis and HIV/Aids combined.
(BBC)

Asthma rates have doubled in Europe in the last ten years.
(UCB Institute of Allergy in Belgium)

20 per cent of children in Kenya now have asthma and between 15 and 20 million children aged five to 11 in India have the condition.
(BBC)

Dental experts in Leeds say the powdered asthma drugs inhaled by increasing numbers of children are sufficiently acidic to dissolve the enamel surfaces of teeth.
(BBC)

'House dust mites can actually cause asthma in the first place'
(National Asthma Campaign's *Asthma News, 2000*)

In the recent Asthma Insights and Reality in Europe (AIRE) survey:

- 73 per cent of asthmatics felt that there was a greater need for patient education.
- 63 per cent of patients said that asthma symptoms limited their activities, including household chores, sports and even choice of jobs. 17 per cent of adults and 43 per cent of children had missed work or school.
- Over 50 per cent of surveyed patients had never received a lung function (e.g. peak flow) test.
- 40 per cent had severe persistent asthma, yet reported that they had their condition well or completely under control.

(European Surveys – Differences in Quality of Life? William C Maier)

The number of disability-adjusted life years lost to asthma worldwide has been estimated at 15 million per year (1 per cent of all the days lost to illness).
(Global Burden of Asthma report, GINA)

Allergy affects about 1 in 3 of the EU population at some time in their lives. Overall, the provision of consultant allergists is 1 per 2 million of the population. Children bear the brunt of allergic disease. In 13 to 14 year old children, 32 per cent report symptoms of asthma, 9 per cent have eczema and 40 per cent have rhinitis.

The UK ranks the highest in the world for asthma.
('Allergy, the unmet need,'
Royal College of Physicians Report, June 2003)

We Are Control Freaks!

The amazing thing about asthma and allergy treatment is that it centres around control. Doesn't sound that amazing.. but hang on... Why don't we try to PREVENT the asthma and allergy?

What we are doing is allowing ourselves to get sick, then taking drugs to control our symptoms - instead of trying not to get sick in the first place.

That's like eating a rotten piece of meat, feeling ill and having to seek medical attention, instead of just eating fresh meat. And doing it again and again.

What could be the cause of this type of thinking?

It's probably the simple result of a lack of education. It's no surprise that your average Joe is not particularly interested in allergy and asthma. Doctors and scientists may know about the allergens that cause you miserable symptoms, but somewhere down the line somebody says 'that's boring' (or 'not lucrative') and the information flow stops before it gets to our schools. So if Average Joe later develops asthma, or has a child with eczema, as a result of his living environment, how is he supposed to know what's going on?

Joe visits the doctor and the doctor prescribes drugs to reduce the body's reactions to allergens. Sounds OK. But the busy doctor will not be able to take an afternoon off to visit Joe's house and teach him how to reduce the allergens. Joe doesn't think his house needs extra cleaning, or even consider that a mild wheezing attack when he's near the cat will affect his future health – he just thinks it's an inconvenience.

So Joe takes the drugs and continues life as a sick person on medication. Because he is IN THE DARK. Joe's kids may even grow up on medication and never kick a ball around because they are 'sickly'.

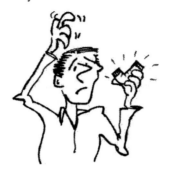

And the weirdest things about this way of thinking are:

- that it's costing us billions to pay for the 'free' medication we are given
- that our societies have been keener to promote drug use than encourage health education at school
- that it passes down from generation to generation without people saying 'hang on, what's in this inhaler/cream/pill? I'd rather not need it!'
- that we unhesitatingly give drugs to our children....

Positive Progress?

Maybe another reason for this obsession with medication, rather than prevention, is connected to the idea that progress is always positive. For example, we are pretty smug about the way we live compared to, say, seventy years ago. In the western world, we now have very comfortable furnishings and central heating, double glazed windows, food that lasts for months, cars that everyone can afford to run, computers and TVs in every home, fast food available where ever you go, international cuisine, etc, etc. I'd hate to be without any of this, to be honest, but it's still fairly obvious that 'modern epidemics' like asthma and obesity are linked to these lifestyle changes.

In the Global Burden of Asthma report from The Global Initiative for Asthma (GINA) it was found that the rate of asthma was increasing as western lifestyles were adopted and the world was becoming more urbanised. The report predicts that, if we keep going this way, we will see 100 million additional asthmatics by 2025. It could be the difference in home furnishings, or fresh, seasonal food.. you are entitled to your opinion, but the stats are there.

It's beginning to sound very depressing but actually, the reason you picked up this book is that you don't want to just accept the 'trend' and go along with this epidemic. You want to know if there's something you can do about it. There is. We survived perfectly happily with less 'stuff' (and more natural pastimes and foods) in the past. We can adapt to, and be content with, all sort of different lifestyles. Just look at the way that the human race has accepted that a great chunk of its population will have to suffer breathing problems! Turn it on its head and think positive - you *can* get used to the simple changes that will help your health.

The modern way of looking at illness tends to be that it's easier to pop a pill than stop using the car for short journeys, or have fresh air flowing round the house, or even cook fresh vegetables instead of a microwave meal.

An excuse is bound to be that we have less time that we used to. For working parents I can see the point. But if you or your children are sensitive and you don't make time to eliminate allergens from your lives, how much more time (and money) are you going to spend dealing with being ill?

The Place For Medicine

I believe we rely on control rather than on prevention because we don't know what causes our illnesses or much about them.

But I am NOT saying there is no place for medicine. Of course there is. Most of us, unfortunately, will need to take medication at certain stages of our life.

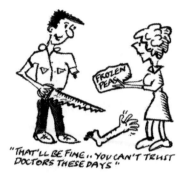

"THAT'LL BE FINE... YOU CAN'T TRUST DOCTORS THESE DAYS"

One important step towards taking control of your health is to understand why you have been prescribed something, instead of just taking it. You will find valuable information about medication in the Global Initiative for Asthma (GINA) booklet for physicians and nurses, 'Pocket Guide for Asthma Management and Prevention in Children', which can be downloaded from the website listed at the back of the book.

Doctors and scientists are often doubtful about 'alternative therapies', because they have not been extensively tested and proven effective, whereas medicines have. The reason for this is largely that pharmaceutical companies fund the research into medicines so that they can market them.

In the Global Burden of Asthma report, the summary lists the main barriers in reducing asthma.

The barriers to asthma patients include:

- cultural factors
- lack of information
- lack of self management
- over-reliance on acute care
- and the use of unproven alternative therapies

I smell a paradox. How are we supposed to manage ourselves and stop relying on acute care if we are not to explore other routes and alternative therapies?

How Your Doctor Should Help You

1. Monitoring your lung function

When you are diagnosed with asthma, you should be asked to blow into a peak flow meter at the doctor's office. This measures your Peak Expiratory Flow, or how well air moves through the passages in your lungs. You might be prescribed a peak flow meter to use at home, with a chart to record the readings on. If not, you can buy one from your local chemist or drug store. This is the easiest way to prove whether or not your asthma is under control.

To use the peak flow meter, breathe out hard into it three times and record your highest reading. This needs to take place every day, morning and night. When there are lower readings it means that your muscles are tightening up, so the diameter of the airways has decreased. That could mean you've been doing something, or been in contact with something, that triggers your asthma off. (This process is explained in the next chapter.) For example, a tall male, aged 30, may have a best peak flow reading of about 650 litres per minute. If he can only puff 450 litres per minute one day, this means that he is at about 70 per cent peak flow, which indicates a mild asthma attack. Easy sums will help you know exactly where you are with your symptoms.

2. Allergen avoidance advice

In conjunction with the peak flow monitoring, you should have been given advice about allergen avoidance (staying clear of things you react to). You will probably have received medication, in the form of an inhaler or possibly a course of steroids. The doctor will want to know how these impact your breathing. The peak flow meter will help you and the doctor or nurse to assess the efficacy of the drugs and any changes in your environment or lifestyle.

If you keep a diary you will be able to make your own assessments about why your asthma improves or gets worse. For example, you might spot a pattern that you get a tight chest after going to a certain friends house, or that there are times of the year that you are more susceptible, or even that stress plays a part. This is a good bit of detective work, as you will get to know exactly what your 'triggers' are. There is now a software package you can use to help you keep proper records (for yourself and your doctor), called 'Asthmalyser'. Have a look at www.sbsoftwaresystems.com if you are interested. For an old fashioned pen and paper template, turn to the back of the book.

3. Medication

Your doctor should tell you what you are taking and what it does (usually you will have medication for preventing asthma long term, as well as for 'rescuing' you when an asthma attack happens.) The doctor or nurse should also demonstrate to you exactly how to take your medicine and make sure that you can use it effectively. You must make sure that you leave the doctor or nurse absolutely confident about what has been prescribed and how you will live with it.

Take Action!

If you are already taking drugs to control asthma, take five minutes now to write down:
1. How often you are supposed to take each type of medicine.
2. The active ingredients of your medications.
3. How they work with your body.
4. What the side effects are.

What, you don't know?!

Every single medicine you take, for asthma or anything else, needs to be taken properly. If you take too much you could damage yourself. You and you doctor should be aiming for life enhancement and a reduction in the amount of medication you need.

Take Action!

1. Find out which drugs you are taking (or about to take).
2. Find out what they do.
3. Research their side effects – they will probably have plenty.
4. Find out about other forms of therapy.

Aim to cut down your medication.

"Drugs are set to rise by 35 per cent in 2011. Better management is called for, not more drugs."
(A quote from Martyn Partridge, medical advisor to Asthma UK, The Sunday Times, 'Style', Feb 22, 2004)

Control And Prevention Together

It would be foolish to distrust what doctors and scientists say and prescribe. However, it is your right and responsibility to maximise prescribed treatments and find out more about your illness.

For example, if my doctor tells me I have a liver disease and prescribes me medicine, then I go home, take the medicine and continue to drink booze like a fish, whose fault is it that my health continues to decline?

It would partly be the doctor's fault, if he had failed to tell me that my liver processes alcohol and could not do so anymore. He would be passively encouraging my ignorance.

But if I knew alcohol was virtually a poison to me and did not avoid it, I might as well drink cyanide for all the good my medicine can do.

In the same vein, if you know that your old mattress and pillows are a haven for house dust mites and that you are inhaling something your body is allergic to every night, do you carry on sleeping in that environment? Relying on your inhaler more and more, instead of changing your bed and taking the inhaler less and less?

Loads of people do.

Your medicine can really help **if** you make lifestyle changes. These are the key to getting better.

Chapter Two

KNOW THE ENEMY!

Your Breathing
Apparatus

"When you have asthma, two things are happening in your lungs.
Constriction is the tightening of the muscles around the airways.
Inflammation is the swelling and irritation of your airways.

Constriction and inflammation both cause narrowing of the airways, which results in wheezing, coughing, a tight chest and breathlessness. There is evidence that untreated asthma can cause long-term decline in lung function."

You'll probably find that sort of description is common on the big web sites you've read about asthma. It's correct, but it gives you a very limited insight. It keeps you on the victim list with Average Joe. You might prefer to know what's going on in a bit more detail.

The respiratory system is a series of tubes and chambers made up of the mouth, nose, windpipe (trachea), and the bronchial tree and alveoli inside the lungs. It looks like an upside-down tree. In an adult, the area of delicate tissue that make up the lungs can be half the size of a tennis court, and all of it is sensitive to what you breathe in.

The trachea and bronchial tree carry the air we breathe into tiny alveoli sacs. This is where the oxygenation of the blood takes place. If this process doesn't happen effectively there may be an imbalance in the exchange between oxygen and carbon dioxide. You exhale carbon dioxide as a waste product. It's vitally important for every cell in your body that the blood that passes through is properly oxygenated, so keeping the balance right is essential. In asthma, swelling of lung tissue and lots of mucous blocking the small airways can cause a gas imbalance.

There is a strong layer of cartilage around the bronchial tubes. Beneath that is a layer of smooth muscle and innermost is the layer that produces mucous, keeping everything 'well-oiled'. Tiny hairs called cilia keep the mucous moving along (and with it the things you breath in that you don't need, like pollen, dog dander, dust mite droppings, etc.)

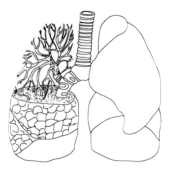

The Lungs

In normal lungs, the muscles around the airways are loose and relaxed and the lining is very thin. This helps the airways to open very wide, allowing air into the sacs for oxygenation.

In all of us, the cilia and smooth muscle may sometimes react to strong smells, smoke or dust, but usually we can breathe freely. In allergy, the immune system within the bronchial tree is always on alert to react.

In an asthmatic lung these muscles have become enlarged and lining of the airways has become swollen or thickened. Because of this, the muscles are always 'twitchy' or sensitive. Just like having a sore, swollen finger, when every little touch hurts like hell. The muscles tighten up and doctors refer to this as **bronchoconstriction,** a common occurrence for asthmatics. Wheezing noises happen when your airflow is disrupted by travelling through narrowed, wonky airways. This turbulence makes a sound – think of organ pipes.

Meet Your Immune Army

We all breathe in foreign particles and allergens that alert our immune defences, but in a normal lung, it's as if the local bobby just politely asks them to move along. And they do, sliding off in the mucous that protects the lung tissue. In an asthmatic's lung, instead of the nice policeman protecting the neighbourhood, the soldiers are straight out with their machine guns, trashing the place at the first sign of a new presence on their patch.

A healthy, mature and balanced immune system is ready to fight dangerous bacterial infections or invasion by parasites as events happen. When the immune system is out of balance, problems can occur. Allergic disease is one example of an imbalanced immune response, but with a little effort it can be controlled.

Upon 'attack' by an allergen (like breathing in dust), the Immunoglobulin E, or IgE, immune system response decides it's a good idea for the airways to spasm, tighten up and try to force the 'invader' (dust) out. The IgE antibodies are present and on the look out because of a previous exposure to the allergen that they have decided is an enemy.

IgE antibodies send Mast cells into the affected area, and these Mast cells spew out all sorts of chemicals to attack the 'invader'.

Type 2 helper T cells, known as Th2, in your blood stream also react to the allergen 'invader'. Th2 fires out loads of chemicals that, as well as killing invading bacteria, will harm and swell up your delicate lung tissue.

Together, these inflammatory cells are the guards of your lung walls. In their heavy arsenal of weapons are chemicals like histamine, endothelin-1, interferon, prostaglandins, bradykinin and leukotrienes.

In allergic people, the body fights allergens with weapons designed for killing parasites. Imagine using a bazooka to kill a rabbit – these weapons are way too powerful for the job of dealing with allergens.

Histamine is the best known of the chemicals used by the immune system as a deadly weapon. It's the overload of histamine that causes us problems, for example itchy eyes in hay fever, or a swollen, itchy reaction to an insect bite. So when you get these symptoms, remember it is the body's overreaction, not the bite or external element, that is the real trouble.

If histamine is just one of an array of chemicals available, consider the damage that can be done to your body's delicate tissue when under full attack. Not only are the chemicals powerful, but they can be delivered long after the allergen has alarmed the immune system. It is this fact that often confuses people. Long after they have been exposed to allergens, an allergic reaction can still occur!

Free Radicals

The inflammatory cells (IgE, Mast, Th2 and others) that come rushing to the scene of any invasion also fire out oxygen molecules called free radicals, which destroy germs and kill any foreign organisms in the body.

In a healthy lung, although the free radicals leave tissue damage where the infection happened, the inflammatory cells will calm down and leave the scene eventually. Our levels of antioxidants - selenium dependant glutathione peroxidase and vitamins A, C and E - will allow our bodies to deal with the effects of free radicals. Not so in the asthmatic lung. Here, the cells are constantly on alert and continue to fire out the chemicals that constrict the muscles in the airways, making them sensitive. Natural antioxidant defences are not enough. Adding to the discomfort experienced in asthma, excessive mucous may have been produced in the airways as a reaction to an allergen – so you're even more bunged up.

Furthermore, your epithelium, the protective lining of your lungs, is spooked by the inflammatory cells into releasing its own chemical weapons – but it damages itself and can break down in places, leaving raw lung tissue exposed.

Yowch!

Asthma Attack!

If you are exposed to an allergen or 'trigger', or if you have not taken your preventer medication to 'numb' your immune system, your army of inflammatory cells is going to leap into action at the first sign of invasion.

A muscle spasm, or asthma attack in the lungs contracts the enlarged airways, making it difficult to breathe out. The air is trapped inside the alveoli sacs. The spasm happens because the muscles 'think' an allergen has been inhaled. With one big effort, they slam shut, hoping to force the object out. This is when you will want your medication urgently, to relax those muscles and restore breathing.

The more often the immune response does this to your lungs, the thicker and more gnarled your airways get. You'll hear this, often, in wheezing. This means that your asthma attacks (you can relate this to other allergic responses too) could get worse over time, if you continue to expose your body to the thing it doesn't like, even in small quantities.

This is why it's important that you don't just rely on preventer steroids to put the immune army to sleep, but instead let it breathe a little fresh air, stop annoying it and help it to relax. Just like letting a wound breathe and recover instead of constantly picking off the scab....

Your body will look after you if you give it the right environment and treat it properly.

The Steps of Asthmatic Reaction

1. Early Allergy Reaction (EAR) is the initial bronchial response **after** 'triggers' or allergens have been inhaled. Chemicals are released by your immune defences, causing inflammation, swelling and the production of excess mucus in the airways. This reaction could happen any time from 30 minutes to two hours after inhalation. Symptoms experienced may be coughing, wheezing or tightness of the chest.

2. Late Allergic Reaction (LAR) may follow EAR as the initial chemicals call upon 'back up' to help them battle against the allergens. This is especially likely to happen if more allergens are inhaled. This reaction takes place any time from 12 to 24 hours after the first exposure. Further damage may be caused as the reaction escalates. The helpers heighten susceptibility to inhaled irritants, such as cigarette smoke, causing the third and seemingly continuous reaction, bronchial hyper responsiveness.

3. Bronchial Hyper Responsiveness (BHR) may come from continuous or repeated exposure of the sensitised lungs to allergens. This leads to chronic symptoms that must be medically treated. Now, muscle contraction can be a real problem, as the lung lining is so tender that it can 'twitch' and contract involuntarily.

So, the lungs of an asthmatic are a bit like an occupied war zone. Foreigners will be treated with suspicion and battles are commonplace. In a non-asthmatic, the lungs are a groovy place where hobos can travel through unnoticed.

If a 'sensitised' (or allergy-prone) lung comes into contact with an invading allergen, it has a whole army of immune cells and chemicals to fight the invasion. We all have a very sensitive immune system, but in many people it is over sensitive, and can cause your body tissues harm as it rages in battle against allergens.

When you avoid breathing in those things that your body gets so worked up about you are giving your immune defences a well-earned rest.

Developing Allergy

Why are some people allergic?

Children who suffer from allergies tend to have a family history of asthma, eczema or rhinitis (hay fever). These unlucky individuals are 'genetically predisposed' or 'Atopic' and are more likely to become allergic than the majority of the population.

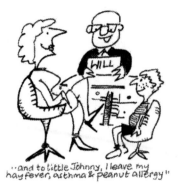

"...and to little Johnny, I leave my hay fever, asthma & peanut allergy"

Atopic asthmatics often have raised levels of IgE - the highly alert immune army lookout that can start an explosive and damaging chemical response to an allergen.

Adult 'late on-set' asthma is not always atopic or to do with the IgE response. In late on-set asthmatics, the immune response is slightly different. The disease, the drugs and the triggers can all be the same, but the immune mechanisms and their response are different. Perhaps hormones, age and the environment have played a role in making the difference. It's a million dollar question.

The term for becoming allergic is to be 'sensitised', or grow sensitive to something in the environment, often a protein from food, animals or plants.

How babies develop immune defence

Some of the early proteins that are thought to cause eczema have been found floating around in the fluid surrounding unborn children. Among these have been elements from mite droppings and a chemical from cigarette smoke, which are both a problem for asthmatics. The presence of them in the womb is a result of the mother's lifestyle and environment. Some babies' immune systems actually recognise these invasive elements at birth – that means they have already been exposed to them and their immune systems have made the decision that these things are not welcome.

Most babies at birth have a defence system looking for invasive parasites such as worms. This defensive reaction is the same mechanism used in later life in an allergic reaction, the Th2 response. (Th means the 'defence' or safeguard' has come from the baby's **Thyroid** gland.)

Following birth, babies 'test' their environment and react to it using their defence systems. There are two major kinds of reactions used in this process; Th1 and Th2. They work together to stop 'invaders' from the environment harming the baby's health.

Th1 mainly fights bacterial infection. Th2 detects and kills parasites. Think of them on either end of a seesaw.

When most babies are born, their body's defence system leans towards a Th2 response. After birth, to maintain good health, the defence mechanisms should balance out, so that Th1 and

Th2 responses are almost equal. This means that the defence systems will recognise parasites and bacteria with equal importance, treating them appropriately.

Usually this is fine; the baby is exposed to various bacteria and so develops a healthy Th1 response. This is an important development in the immune system which can take up to eight years to fully mature.

But some babies appear to be slow in making this change and establishing the right balance. They might, therefore, get locked into a Th2 type of response. This imbalance means that the Th2 response will be working overtime, mistakenly recognising proteins (allergens) as parasites. The result of this could be allergy.

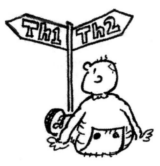

Why Th2 is a problem

Say a flea bites you. Once the Th2 response has recognised a protein from the insect as an enemy, it calls for chemicals within the body to be released to destroy the protein and an itchy bump may appear. If you are allergic, and this recognised 'enemy protein' or allergen has entered the body, the Th2 may also target your delicate tissues around the allergen, damaging you. The damage is usually inflammation, or swelling. When a foreign protein enters the lungs, you may start to feel and hear the breathing problems associated with asthma. The Th2 immune response has caused problems by over reacting. The trouble is that it gets into a habit of over reacting to quite innocent visitors, and starts to recognise more and more proteins from the environment as troublemakers. It's a bit like an over protective guard dog.

In the early years of life, the proteins that may encourage this kind of reaction from Th2 are from foods such as egg whites, milk, wheat and fish. The inhaled proteins that cause reactions at this time are from house dust mites, furry pets, cockroaches and moulds.

The first signs of allergy

One of the first indications of a problem with allergy may start with a skin condition known as allergic dermatitis or eczema. Eczema can be the result of the body's defence system attacking a protein it thinks is an invader, just like the asthma attack.

This attack involves a release of chemicals that cause the red, itchy blotches that are the hallmark of the condition. Itchiness and scratching break the skin's barrier and make the area sore. Doctors refer to eczema as 'the itch that erupts, not the eruption that itches'. Once the skin is broken there is obviously more danger of infection, or entry by other proteins and bacteria. The defence system is always ready to recognise any new invaders that it thinks may threaten your health. Eczema is one of the earliest indications of allergy that could lead to asthma, from triggers like dust, pets and food. It may also be linked to stress, as the cells that produce the 'itch' are closely related to nerve endings in the body.

Chronic rhinitis (runny or blocked nose) is a known risk factor for the development of asthma and should be controlled. If it is seasonal, it's usually known as hay fever. However, perennial rhinitis, when you have symptoms all year round, is likely to be an allergy to the indoor environment.

A constant runny or bunged-up nose is usually a tell-tale sign that an allergy is at the bottom of the problem.

Various events later in life, such the hormonal changes of puberty may help your immune army (including Th2) forget its habitual response – you may outgrow it. However, once you have been diagnosed as allergic or atopic, you should be on your guard.

There is research going on constantly, discovering how allergy can be predicted, or how the environment plays a part in the disease. It is thought by many that genes and the environment are equal partners in allergy.

Nobody is prepared to stand up and say, 'This is what causes asthma', as there are far too many variables. But scientists working for Asthma UK (formerly the National Asthma Campaign) quietly acknowledged in 2000 that 'The house dust mite can actually cause asthma in the first place.' That was a major breakthrough in their research... Anyway, the studies continue but, to me, the temptation to link our modern levels of asthma with our modern environment is just too compelling to ignore! That means that it's within our control.

All About Mites

Mites are survivors!

Fossil studies show that mites have been on earth for over 400 million years.

It is estimated that today there may be up to 100 million different species of mites in existence, from the bottom of the ocean to the most remote desert. They have even been extracted from blocks of Tundra ice.

Some mites have peculiar habitats, including the windpipe of a bee, the ear of a moth or the hair follicle on a human's face.

There are dozens of types of storage mite, among them 'Lepidoglyphus destructor', found in poorly stored organic products at home (like bags of flour) and Acarus Silo, which lives in UK grain stores – and about 90 per cent of this type are now immune to insecticides!

Ticks are just big mites.

The Oribatid mite is a secondary decomposer of soil, and the humus it helps from is vital for plant growth.

If this has tickled your fancy, read more in 'Aracology, Mites and Human Welfare' by TA Wooley (ISBN-0-470-04618-8).

House dust mites

The house dust mite (HDM) evolved 23 million years ago as a scavenger living in birds' nests or similar habitats. Approximately 10,000 years ago mites discovered the human environment, which has got cosier and cosier for it over time.

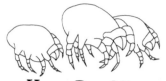

House Dust Mites

'Dermatophagoides pteronyssissinus' is the posh name for the HDM normally found in Europe. Its cousin 'Dermatophagoides farinae' is more common in the USA. All HDMs have eight legs, each with a sucker and hooks. This ensures easy travel on clothing, blankets, soft toys and old furniture - to colonise and infest suitable nest sites if the conditions are right. The conditions needed are warm, dark and damp. Perfect conditions would be 73 per cent relative humidity and temperatures of around 25 degrees centigrade.

The HDM is unable to regulate its body temperature, has no eyes, no organised respiratory system and its body weight is up to 80 per cent water. It absorbs water and air through its outer shell. Maturity from egg to adult may take up to 30 days in a life-span of approximately three months, depending upon living conditions and sex of the mite. Females can lay up to 100 eggs and live slightly longer than males. Amazingly, the females can store sperm until her eggs are ready. The mites are too small to be seen with the naked eye, at about 0.4 mm.

The HDM lives mainly on fungi and rotting skin scales, but as a scavenger it will eat what is available. Human skin scales are approximately ten per cent fat and too rich for the mite when freshly shed – the HDM prefers a meal that's been hanging around a while, so eats the skin once mould has had a chance to break it down. This mould is nourishing for the mite too, and is present in its droppings.

The mite creates up to 20 dung pellets a day. These droppings, which are devoid of moisture and wrapped in a special film, contain scraps of food, debris and powerful enzymes. The enzymes continue to break down any remaining food (skin) particles; thus ensuring nourishment for the mite later. In other words they can eat their own poo up to three times over.

The mite's microscopic dung pellets, if disturbed in an unventilated room, can remain suspended in still air for 20 minutes. During this time they can be easily inhaled by unsuspecting people.

Why house dust mites are a problem

As long ago as 1662 it was realised that the inhalation of dust particles in the air led to symptoms of allergic reaction. In the 1920s, German doctor Dekker designed a bed to eliminate mites. Not until 1981 did doctors establish the HDM element Der p1 as a major cause of allergy in house dust.

We now know that a huge 85 per cent of asthmatics are allergic to the house dust mite.

There are 16 known allergens from the HDM. Derp2 is thought to come from the mite's genital tract or immune system. Another major allergen, Der p1, in the droppings is so invasive that it has been found in foetal amniotic fluid at 16-17 weeks gestation and in the cord blood of some babies at birth.

Doctors have found that Der p1 causes the breakdown the molecules that bind the cells of the lung, causing little holes in the cell walls and a breach of the lung's defence system. (Remember, these enzymes are designed to break down human skin cells to make them more digestible to mites.) This means cell death, leaving other cells more exposed to inhaled allergens or micro-organisms (fungi and bacteria). Potentially harmful bacterial micro-organisms have been found living in the airways of adults with chronic asthma.

Once in the lung, the enzymes in the HDM droppings continue to break down specific molecules. The over-sensitive immune system thinks that this is an invasion and reacts with a spasm to protect itself. This should move the allergen away through the airways, but the tight, constricted tubes and thick mucous mean that the HDM droppings can hang around and do damage in asthmatic lungs.

In short, house dust mites lead to asthma attacks, and asthma attacks lead to lung damage. That's why we consider it important that people should be more aware of the effects of house dust mites.

As the cherry on the cake, if inhaled allergens like dust mite droppings are accompanied by chemicals from cigarette smoke or excessive ozone, the activity of the mite's allergens can be amplified. The chemicals lessen the ability of lungs to defend the body from aggressive allergens such as pollens, moulds and mites, making them even more dangerous than nature intended.

Take Action!

If you have kids or prefer to learn about this through animations, please have a look at www.housedustmite.org.

Other Allergens

Apart from the house dust mite, you may need to look out for some other triggers around you. Keeping a simple diary of what you've eaten and, most importantly, where you've been, will help you to find out what you need to avoid – remember, if you suddenly get asthma symptoms for no apparent reason, then they are probably 'stored up' from something you did earlier. You need to do some detective work here. There's an example of a very 'simple but effective' diary template at the back of this book.

The 'wheel of misfortune' over the page shows the major allergen groups (and influences, which are not allergens but can exacerbate breathing problems) and below that is a list of the most common troublemakers.

Remember, although lots of people say that they are allergic to some foods, this is not always true. They probably mean that they are intolerant. Pets, mould and other allergens are much more likely to be the real source of allergy problems in people over ten years old.

The Wheel of Misfortune

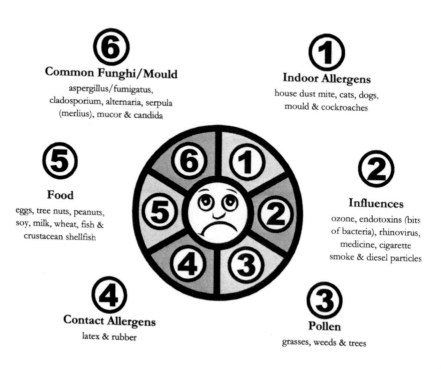

⑥ Common Funghi/Mould
aspergillus/fumigatus, cladosporium, alternaria, serpula (merlius), mucor & candida

① Indoor Allergens
house dust mite, cats, dogs, mould & cockroaches

⑤ Food
eggs, tree nuts, peanuts, soy, milk, wheat, fish & crustacean shellfish

② Influences
ozone, endotoxins (bits of bacteria), rhinovirus, medicine, cigarette smoke & diesel particles

④ Contact Allergens
latex & rubber

③ Pollen
grasses, weeds & trees

The usual suspects

Cats

Skin and saliva from cats are a big cause of problems in allergy. The protein that causes trouble is called Fel d1. This is a double strand protein made up of many different components. Not every allergic person is sensitive to the same combination of components in the protein. This can cause problems for doctors trying to ascertain whether or not you are allergic to cats with the skin prick test.

People who have never even lived with a cat can develop an allergy to them, because the allergens are particularly invasive. Even in a place with no resident or visiting cats, the cat proteins are present. It's probably because the allergens stick to the cat's fur, which then sticks to its owners, goes everywhere they go and ends up sticking to everything. All cat owners will sympathise that this is definitely the case. The complex cat allergens are still under the scrutiny of scientists.

Cockroaches

Cockroach body parts, saliva (urgh) and droppings are allergenic. Stay away.. don't be tempted to live with these cuddly creatures. The protein is called Bla g4. Cockroaches cause asthma problems in inner cities or in dry and arid climates.

Cow's milk

Bovine Serum Albumin in moo juice has been known to penetrate the gut of an infant and raise allergic antibodies, leading to overactive allergic response. However, cows milk is also the most important source of calcium for strong bones, so don't avoid it unless you absolutely have to according to a medical specialist.

Dogs

Dander (dust from fur), skin and saliva are recognised allergens from dogs. Their dander is a big problem for adults with eczema. Proteins called Can f1 and Can f2 come from these allergens and they can cause an IgE response in allergic people. And would you believe, Can f2 is found in mouse urine too. Doggy dander can float about in a room for two to four hours before it settles.

Eggs

Allergy to egg white is often the first allergy developed in childhood. Peptides, which are protein-like molecules in the egg white, bind to tissue cells, causing them to release the chemicals associated with allergic reaction.

False food allergy

Strawberries, shellfish, eggs, tomatoes and some fish are in a category of foods that can trigger the Mast cell response but are nothing to do with the usual IgE allergic response associated with food.

Fish

Bony white fish, like cod, have a protein called parvalbumin that can trigger allergy in some people. The dominant allergen is called Gad a1. Usually, fish is a very important part of a healthy diet.

Funghi

The funghi 'Aspergillus fumigatus' can colonise in the lung, causing alveolitis. It can grow in mattresses and around the house. Other moulds and funghi can be a problem in the autumn, or year-round in damp houses. Fungal toxins are not allergenic, but can pose problems for sensitive lungs.

Histamine

Formed in food by harmless bacteria. For some people, ripe cheese, continental sausages, mackerel, tuna, tinned fish, sauerkraut and alcohol, which can all contain histamine, may cause a reaction. The reaction could be flushed skin, an itchy rash, a headache, nausea, diarrhoea or chronic urticaria. It's rare, because usually your enzymes can break down histamine, even in large quantities.

Latex – rubber

Some people might find they have to stay clear of rubber gloves. Could be problematic for surgeons, those dealing with chemicals and in many other scenarios. The powder in some gloves can absorb latex, which can then puff off into the atmosphere. Watch what you cover your mattresses in.

Mould

A mould called 'Alternaria' is known to cause asthma symptoms. It's commonly found on cultivated plants.

Medicine

Some asthmatics will be asked to avoid aspirin – it can lead to the overproduction of leukotrienes (part of your immune army's OTT chemical weaponery that can cause you problems). Penicillin may need to be avoided and all asthmatics should steer clear of beta-blockers.

Ozone O3

Ozone comes from thunderstorms, ultraviolet light, some photocopiers and car exhaust fumes. It's an unstable toxic gas that reacts with respiratory tissue.

Peanuts

Children suspected to be atopic should not have peanuts before the age of seven. After that, many people find they can introduce peanuts to their diet. However, be careful, as this allergy can cause nasty skin and breathing problems, or even anaphylaxis.

Soy

Like a peanut, soy is from a legume (pod of a plant, pea or bean) and rich in lectin. Lectin is a group of proteins found mainly in plant seeds and it binds to the branching sugar molecules on the surface of cells. This may cause clumping and leaky gut, letting particles of undigested food through to the blood stream. This can raise the IgE antibodies that over react in allergy. Make sure you cook beans and chick peas thoroughly.

Traffic fumes

Nitrogen Dioxide and other air pollutants found in traffic fumes affect many asthmatics. Diesel engines produce these more than petrol engines, and many cities have twice the acceptable level as defined by the World Health Organisation. Diesel particles are also able to 'piggy back' proteins and when these are absorbed on the diesel particle's surface, they can become more allergenic.

Wheat germ

Similar to the peanut in the way it can clump. The major allergen here is thought to be alpha-amlase inhibitor, but wheat allergy is pretty rare in adults. Usually, wheat is something that people with Irritable Bowel Syndrome have intolerance to.

Finding Out What You're Allergic To

Lots of eczema, asthma and rhinitis sufferers know that they have a 'condition' but never enquire about what causes it. Or, even if they know that they are reacting to certain allergens like to the house dust mite's droppings, they assume that they just have to live with the little beasties. This is one situation where ignorance definitely does NOT equal bliss.

Once you begin to find out more about what makes you react, you will become more powerful to fight the things that your body hates.

Your doctor can advise you on allergy testing. Once symptoms of allergy have been recognised, whether they are gut problems, asthma, eczema or hay fever, a doctor may be able to identify your triggers by giving you a 'skin prick' test. Samples of various allergens are placed on your arm or back and any resulting red mark (mini reaction) will identify a trigger. Blood samples may be taken to perform the same test. These tests are not conclusive or 100 per cent reliable, but are very useful indicators. The doctor will then be able to advise what you should avoid and prescribe you the proper medicine, if appropriate.

Many doctors recommend that patients who suspect they have a food intolerance do an 'elimination diet'. You will be able to find self help books about this, but a simple way to do it is identify the food groups, such as lactose (milk, cheese), wheat (bread, cereals), etc and just do seven days without one group until you feel better or your symptoms decrease. Speaking from experience of doing this, the improvement you feel can be enormous, so it's definitely worth investigating.

Using this method of discovering food intolerance is also helpful in dealing with allergy. You can treat the house dust mite as a food group (after all, that's what it does to you). Try to avoid contact with the mite's droppings for a while. The ways to do this are listed in Chapter Four.

Is Asthma Really That Serious?

You already know that asthma is a disease that can lower your quality of life. But, have you thought about the 'knock-on effects'?

Here are just a few:

People who suffer with allergy and asthma tend to miss more work or school than average through sickness.

People with asthma often suffer with acute tiredness because of their coughing at night. They then under perform at school and work.

Children with allergy and asthma are less able to run around with their healthier counterparts, and don't build up their strength, fitness and bodily defences as effectively as a result.

Those who suffer with chronic asthma in childhood are much more likely to be sick throughout their adult life. They may have lung damage and poor bodily defences for fighting off disease.

Lack of exercise means:

Weaker bones.. Less muscle mass.. More body fat.. A less effective heart.. A less alert mind.. Under performance at work and school.. More time at indoors amongst the allergens.. More allergic reaction.. Less exercise.. Weaker bones.. Less muscle mass...

If you are letting asthma rule your life, it's **very** serious.. Make the changes now!

Chapter Three

THE PILGRIM BED STUDY

The Pilgrim Bed Study

In 1997 the Nockles family designed an educational programme and anti allergen bed for children, drawing on their research and experience.

The bed and bedroom of an asthmatic can cause huge problems. Because they are full of soft furnishings and are dark and damp (we all sweat at night) they are the dust mite's ideal breeding ground. This is why the Nockles' felt that they should tackle the problem by designing a bed that could not harbour mites and mould, but instead promoted clear breathing and airflow.

The Pilgrim Bed and 'sleeping system' realistically combined the lifestyle aspects Nell Nockles had discovered would benefit an asthmatic. The family was convinced that the study they were about to begin could mean enormous health benefits for thousands of allergic asthmatics.

Getting started

In 1998 the medical study to evaluate the effects of the Pilgrim Bed began. East Surrey Health Authority (ESHA) supported the study designed for twenty asthmatic children, with their families, doctors and asthma nurse. The collaboration of all these parties was key in properly evaluating the children's medical progress.

The Pilgrim Bed study programme included the following:

- Educational video by Dr Jill Warner about allergen recognition and avoidance
- Educational booklets
- Air mattress – to prevent mite colonisation

- Pilgrim Bed (designed to promote airflow and to appeal to kids)
- Micro porous pillow covers
- Washable cotton quilted cover for the mattress, designed to absorb sweat and transportable allergens from cats or and dogs.
- Peak flow chart to monitor lung function during the study
- Dehumidifier (for loan to patients)

Educational stuff included games, puzzles, booklets, colouring books and demonstrations of avoidance techniques. All were used considering the age of the child and the potential uptake of information. Other teaching aids came from published papers/graphs and videos demonstrating the effect of allergens upon the asthmatic child.

Advice was given to all the families about how to keep a home well-ventilated, free of dust, clutter and dampness, and about the importance of not letting pets in the child's bedroom. This was done in the patients' homes, by the Nockles family and supported by asthma nurses and doctors.

Most of the houses were so full of allergens that Nell had to stop going on these introductory sessions and keep in contact by phone, as her asthma was being triggered off again. But these were NORMAL, family homes. As they talked to the families, an overall lack of understanding about environmental allergens including allergens from house dust mites, mould and furry pets was noticed. The study found that 75 per cent of the participants kept at least one furry animal of some sort inside the home. 80 per cent were using old non micro-filtration vacuum cleaners and generally re-used the bags. All clues as to why the children's asthma had got so bad.

The Study

The British Thoracic Society says in its guidelines for the 'Management of Chronic Asthma in Adults and Schoolchildren' that **patient involvement and education, avoidance of provoking factors** where possible and **properly controlled medication** are key elements in the management of the disease.

The ESHA study investigated these three elements through the partnership of a General Practitioner's surgery, a children's hospital clinic, the Pilgrim Bed and the educational system.

This was a multi-centred study, designed to promote communication between the home visitor (primary care worker), asthma clinics and the general practitioner or paediatrician.

The study period was 26 weeks, including autumn and winter. The sample population diagnosed as asthmatic and sensitive to the house dust mite was identified from computer and out-patient records. Letters inviting families to participate in the study were sent out to patients of the medical centre.

The sample size was 20 children born between 1st January 1983 and 31st December 1993 (aged between five and 15 years) and consisted of 12 children from the medical centre and nine children from the general hospital.

To be included in the study, children had to have at least one year's diagnosis of asthma, a bedroom to themselves and therapy level at steps two and three (as defined by the British Thoracic Society, see above).

If they were allergic to latex, had a bedroom smaller than eight feet square or couldn't prevent pets getting into the bedroom, they were not allowed to take part in the study.

Once identified by the asthma nurse, the candidates were given the new bed and bedding and the educational programme. This programme, designed to inform and consolidate the message of allergen avoidance, started with a series of home visits by the Nockles. Monitoring of the progress of the child's health and family attitude towards the programme was noted at each visit. A total of 158 home visits were made to the 20 patients.

Parents and guardians appreciated the peak flow monitoring, as it showed how the environment made a difference to the child's asthma and this gave them a trustworthy overview of their child's health progress. This is the same type of peak flow monitoring your doctor should ask you to do when deciding your care plan.

The idea was simple – could asthmatic children be helped just by changing their home and sleep environments? Could medication use be decreased? Could these children experience better quality of life?

If the answer to these questions was yes – could the burden of asthma on our economy and health service be lessened, meaning better funding in other areas?

The Results

Drug usage at the end of the 26 weeks

61 per cent of the children studied had reduced their usage of prescribed reliever
38 per cent had reduced their usage of prescribed inhalers and relievers
33 per cent neither increased or decreased their drug usage
5 per cent had an increase of drug usage during the study period

Attacks and symptoms at the end of the 26 weeks

Results from this study confirm that parents, asthma nurses and doctors found:

✓ **Less acute episodes**
In the report, **acute episodes** were defined as being a worsening of asthma requiring the use of a nebuliser, a short course of oral steroids, a home visit from a GP or hospital admission.

✓ **Improved control of symptoms**
Symptoms were defined as shortness of breath at night, tightness of the chest on waking, exercise-induced symptoms and absenteeism from school.

✓ **Improved compliance with prescribed medication**
This implies that the education programme had an impact on correct drug useage

✓ **No asthma-related full consultative episodes**
A serious **full consultative episode (FCE)** costs the East Surrey Health Authority approximately £1320 per patient.

Over the last few years the annual average has been 500 FCEs in this area. Nationally, one in seven children are diagnosed as asthmatic and 8,000 are children from East Surrey. (1999)

The study improved allergic asthma for most of the children.

Asthma costs the UK over £2 billion per annum. In East Surrey the cost of prescribed medication for asthma is over £4 million per annum.(1999) See the patient feedback for evidence of improved life quality.

✓ **An overall health-gain was shown.**

✓ **The educational programme was appreciated by most families.**

✓ **Most families requested more information on major allergens.**

✓ **Less absenteeism from school was reported**
Asthma is the biggest reason for absenteeism in schools, and is on the increase. Recent years have seen a marked increase in the number of children presenting symptoms of allergic asthma. (1999)

The Pilgrim bed at the end of 26 weeks

Following these results, more Pilgrim Beds and education packs were produced, but they were never successfully marketed to the public. A university student, studying for a Master's degree in marketing, investigated why the Pilgrim Bed had failed to make a mark. The student concluded that the public and medical profession were both sceptical of the need for change in the sleeping environment. Remember the 'control not prevention' school of thought?

The beds are still stacked up in a barn in Wiltshire, but the low allergen sleeping concept has already done its job, as you can see from the results above and comments below. The bed was also given 'Millennium Product' status by the UK's Design Council and recognised by the British Library as a future product of importance. What a shame parents and guardians of asthmatic children never got to hear about it…

Patient Feedback

To give you more idea of the impact of the ESHA and Pilgrim Bed study, please read these comments from the study children's parents. (Names are changed for confidentiality reasons.)

Hopefully you will be inspired – something this simple can have dramatic effects on asthma!

Ajay (aged 9)

"The bed has clearly, positively, affected Ajay's night-time rest. He has not had a disturbed night. This plus the peak-flow shows better breathing. The education process has improved both Ajay's and my understanding of the underlying causes of asthma; an understanding of what happens during an asthma attack; and also how to avoid, or decrease, asthma triggers. In summary, it allows Ajay to be in charge of his asthma, rather than the other way around."

Becky (aged 10)

"Since Becky began to use the Pilgrim Bed she has reduced the amount of reliever she was having to take. She has suffered one bad cold and found that increasing her medication combined with the use of the bed, her symptoms were far more easily controlled than in the past. We have learned that a dry, dust free environment is also greatly beneficial to Becky's health."

Colin (aged 7)

"Colin hasn't had any chest infections since using the Pilgrim Bed and his overall health has been fine. He no longer coughs during the night or on waking up in the morning although his peak-flow record doesn't show much improvement. I have noticed fewer asthmatic symptoms and he has needed his Ventolin inhaler less. I am certain Colin's health has improved since using the bed and he likes it too!"

David (aged 13)

"David has used this bed for approximately 4 months and has slept right through the night virtually from day one. This is something that I didn't think was possible. Going to bed was always a performance of waiting for the cough, then dealing with it (inhalers) then settling him down, then gradually waiting for the coughing to slow down and eventually he would fall asleep, virtually exhausted. David has also had the best peak-flow readings he has ever had and when he wakes in the morning there is no cough! While he has still had his wheezy attacks and his bad days he has never had that terrible cough that I dread to hear. I know it is early days and we still have the winter to get through but I am very pleased with the bed so far and would be very reluctant to give it up."

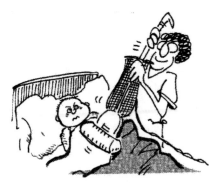

Edward (aged 8)

"I feel the Pilgrim Bed has had an impact on Edward's health. Since having the bed Edward sleeps through the night without waking up coughing which he has done before. The Pilgrim Bed has been a great comfort for me and more so for Edward."

Fiona (aged 9)

"During the course of the study, Fiona's asthma has improved to the extent that she has been able to stop taking Becotide. It is difficult to say how much of this is due to the bed as she has started puberty. As this is a time when asthma often improves it is difficult to know which has had

most effect. Undoubtedly, though, Fiona's knowledge of asthma and potential allergens has increased."

Geraldine (aged 12)

"The combination of the Pilgrim Bed and the health education we have received on the programme have, without doubt, greatly improved Geraldine's condition. The night time coughing Geraldine experienced led us to suspect that her asthma was in some way related to her bedding. We had subsequently replaced her original bedding with hypoallergenic duvet and pillows. The environmental changes we have made since joining the study would not have been considered without the education we have received from Nell. I only regret that this study didn't occur earlier in Geraldine's life thus saving her many years of misery at the hands of asthma."

Harry (aged 7)

"Harry's asthma has improved immensely since the Pilgrim Bed was introduced to us. Although I can't give exact results I would estimate that his school attendance has improved by 95%. The small amount of time he has had off this year was not due to asthma related illness, therefore we are seeing much improvement with school work. I'm sure his teachers would agree.

I can also confirm that we have not visited our GP for antibiotics for chest infections since the bed arrived and have reduced the daily dosage of inhaler. Previously, Harry would have a cold every few weeks, which would end up with a chest infection and would result in antibiotics. He has had a few colds but they have not ended up on his chest.

I think that I can now describe Harry's asthma as under control and have the Pilgrim Bed to thank for such improvement. I now have the confidence to let him go to after-school activities. His busy schedule follows: Football on Tuesdays & Thursdays; Basketball on Wednesdays; Swimming on Tuesdays and Saturdays."

Jean (aged 12)

"Her health is very much better and Jean has not had any time off school, also she sleeps much better."

Keith(aged 7)

"Keith's peak-flow reading has increased from approx. 250 to around 300 since the Pilgrim Bed was installed. It is a cold bed but with very helpful knowledge from Mrs Nockles this was sorted out very quickly. Keith sleeps well and comfortably in the Pilgrim Bed."

Lorna (aged 7½)

"Since Lorna started the programme we have noticed a great difference both in sleep and school. Lorna is now able to have a comfortable night with no coughing and waking up feeling refreshed. When it comes to school Lorna has lost no attendance whereas last year she lost about 21 days. What an improvement! Also she is able to do most P.E. lessons and she has taken up Skipping Club."

Mary (aged 7)

"She is enjoying her bed - sleeping well- and obviously there is no marked progress as yet. Her asthma has not affected her school attendance this term."

Neil (aged 12)

"Thanks to your advice and since the installation of your bed, Neil has not had an asthma attack, with obvious health gain resulting in reduced medication."

Oliver (aged 8½)

"Oliver's benefits from the programme are 1) an increase in his awareness (and his mother's) of the causes and control of asthma through the education process and 2) an improvement in his ability to breathe as demonstrated by the peak-flow chart. This fluctuates more than we would like, so we are closely monitoring and endeavouring to take into account other variables."

Paul (aged 8)

"At present, Paul is symptom-free. This is the longest "good-stretch" with no problems for 4 months although he is still on medication twice daily. Paul feels settled in his new bed and is very happy. Paul has only been on the study for a short while and so far I feel that our more in depth understanding of House Dust Mites and household situations has given us both more confidence to cope. I now feel more in control!"

Queenie (aged 9)

"Less fluctuation in peak-flow readings. This is particularly noticeable when Queenie has a cold or virus and means that she has not needed to take any time off school due to her asthma this term. Her general level of fitness also appears to have improved."

Richard (aged 6)

"Richard has now been on a Pilgrim Bed for 10 weeks. During this time it is our definite view that Richard appears to be more relaxed and less restless during sleep and we believe he coughs less at night. He definitely sneezes less in the mornings. We have learnt from the "Education Programme" and have made several changes to his home environment as identified in the programme. Richard has enjoyed and responded well to the information given to us, also. Whilst being on the programme Richard has had one week off sick from school with a fairly severe throat and respiratory virus. This did cause disturbed nights and his peak flow dropped. However, although poorly, his chest did not appear to be affected. This was confirmed on consultation by the paediatric registrar at Epsom Hospital."

Sarah (aged 10)

"Sarah's asthma awareness has been greatly enhanced by the education she has received whilst being on the programme. She is much more aware of the 'triggers'. Her peak-flow ranges from 300 - 370 so this goes up-and-down, but her asthma seems to be improved, although January appears to be one of her worst months. This next year may be different."

Tom (aged 6)

"We believe that there has been a general improvement in Tom's condition; probably due to the replacement of the mattress and more scrupulous washing of linens, soft toys and clothes. We are complementing the study with alternative medicines to combat his reaction to viral attacks. So far having suffered cold symptoms plus exposure to cats, his reactions have been contained and not developed into asthma."

Vernon and Victor (aged 11 and 13)

Vernon *"The Pilgrim Bed has really helped me with my asthma it's a big success. The bed would certainly help more people like me. Looking at my peak flow it steadily rises all through the study."*

Victor *"The Pilgrim Bed has helped me a lot with stopping me feeling wheezy and short for breath in the morning and it has also taught me a lot about allergens and what asthma does inside you. Doing the study I've found things out like what my triggers are and what to avoid to stay healthy. This is an excellent help for asthmatics and I hope it can help many more people in years to come, it is excellent!"*

From mother of Vernon and Victor *"This would have been invaluable when Vernon was younger, and may even have prevented him attending casualty and having steroids. This is the best winter Vernon has had health-wise, he has had few illness-related events and has fought off colds effectively. Victor is also better but it took longer in his case to identify why his peak flow was low in the mornings even with the bed. Detective work was invaluable here!"*

NB - Xavier and Yolanda were participating in a parallel study in Cambridge

Xavier (aged 7)

"Xavier's general health has been very good since having the bed. He has, so far, had full attendance at school, which is something to be very pleased about. He has not suffered from any allergies or colds so far. Xavier has only been wheezy about four times since we started on the scheme."

Yvonne (aged 8)

"Since Yvonne started using her Pilgrim Bed her overall asthma health has improved. Use of Ventolin has been very limited and usually due to outside effects — someone smoking, certain pets, etc. When we visit certain friends however, we can notice an immediate effect — swollen red eyes, harder breathing, etc. This we put down to the house where people smoke, pets kept indoors. It immediately improves when we get home."

Why you didn't hear about these results

After the study's encouraging results, the NHS made moves towards a larger study to confirm that multi-system allergen avoidance can make a difference in asthma. It was all going well, then one day it stopped. The Nockles family was informed that no money would be available to progress the concept further. Asthma UK (then known as the National Asthma Campaign), the leading information source in asthma, had to continue to focus on drugs as the best treatment for the disease.

The ESHA study was very important to all of us, asthmatic or not. It went some way towards proving that an effective way to tackle one of our most prevalent and expensive diseases is to AVOID ALLERGENS AND TAKE RESPONSIBILITY FOR HEALTH IN THE HOME.

Take action!

Take a moment to consider the great effect allergen avoidance may have on you or your family's health.

Ask yourself why the public has been directed towards drug therapy rather than education.

Read on for the simple solutions that can make all the difference..

Chapter Four

EASY WAYS TO
CHANGE YOUR ENVIRONMENT

Where Are The Trouble Spots?

First, find the enemy. I don't know what your house is like, so get the Sherlock Holmes hat on and start thinking about your home in terms of pet fur, skin cells, humidity, mould, damp washing.. and the dreaded mite.

Because the mite is the one you can't see, feel or smell, it tends to get overlooked. But remember, for 85 per cent of asthma sufferers it is a major culprit! Seeking it out is a question of brainstorming and, if you live with kids, it's a good way for them to really start thinking about allergen avoidance.

e.g. If I tell you that house dust mites love damp or sweaty places, warmth, darkness and a good supply of human skin cells (dust) to eat, where in your house are they most likely to be?

These are all good answers, but keep trying to find more:

Mattress
Duvet
Blankets
Pillows
Cushions
Teddies
Carpets
Rugs
Under and in the sofa
Linen baskets
Linen cupboards
Chairs
Cushions
Thick curtains
Dog baskets

When I say House Dust Mites love these places, I mean these places are crawling. Infested with tiny mites, depositing their eggs and droppings. In a humid, high-allergen environment, the pillows on your bed, damp from your face and the occasional dribble are a perfect breeding ground, right near the entrance to your lungs. If you or your kids are asthmatic, that's bad news.

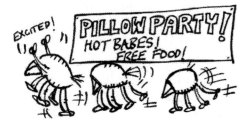

OK, this isn't supposed to freak you out, but the key is to start looking at things in your house as potential dust mite homes. Where are the beasties doing their worst? Get rid of their cosy breeding grounds and stop breathing in the droppings that can damage your lung tissue and have a negative effect on your quality of life.

If you can't get rid of the things that may be nesting sites, you should look into ways of cleaning them that will eliminate the mites and their eggs..

What Could Help
My Home?

Dehumidifiers

Dehumidifiers are fairly easy to get hold of, especially online, and control the amount of moisture in the air. This should be below 50 per cent relative humidity - comfortable for us but a disaster for mite colonies. Humidity at 55 per cent encourages house dust mites to survive, above 60 per cent it encourages them to breed.

Reducing humidity really is the best way to control house dust mite populations, and climatic humidity may be largely to blame for the higher incidence of mite related asthma in damp countries like the UK.

These days, double glazed windows, en suite bathrooms and showers, more pets and more hours spent inside all add to humidity in the house. You can reduce humidity easily, once you are aware of the need to keep it low!

Ventilation

Plenty of fresh air and sunshine are good for you. Same for your house. House dust mites hate both. Vacuum and air your mattress on sunny days with the window open. If you're an asthmatic, get someone to do this for you. Make sure that a window or two are open as much as possible to promote a healthy airflow. The draft will send disturbed allergens outside where they won't cause any harm. This goes for the whole house, especially in rooms with soft furnishings. Pretend you were born in a barn and keep the doors ajar.

Asthma is all about breathing.... And even non-asthmatics should find their energy levels increase with more fresh air around.

Furnishings

If you can get rid of any ancient three piece suites you will eliminate a vast house dust mite city. Choose furniture that is easy to keep clean instead, like wipe clean blinds or easy to wash curtains. Carpets – a contentious issue. On the website, we have often advised that carpets are unhealthy, mite ridden places and that you should opt for lino, tiles or laminate instead. However, I'm now told that if you have a short pile carpet with no underlay, it could be healthier than a smooth floor. This is because, as you walk around, the allergens will tend to stick to the carpet instead of flying about. If you have laminate, for example, those allergens can become suspended in the air (in a poorly ventilated room), where you can breathe them in, or they can transfer to sofas etc. It's the old, soft, thicker pile carpets, in a humid, that are the real problem. No amount of vacuuming can get all the mites and allergens out of these carpets. If you're really stuck with what you have or unwilling to change it, see below.

Sprays

There are various chemical sprays available, which eliminate house dust mites and their eggs from your furniture and carpets. **Be careful** and seek advice when using chemicals. Have you researched all your allergies?

It's best to stick to products that have had the British Allergy Foundation's Seal of Approval.

Insecticides will not work on mites, so please don't try it. Mites come from a different family.

Freezing

Cushions, teddies, pillows.. any smallish object that harbours dust mites will benefit from an overnight stay in the deep freeze, as dust mites and their eggs will be destroyed. Washing, vacuuming or hanging out in the fresh air afterwards will help get rid of the allergens left behind.

Heat treatment

With big items of furniture, washing is not an option. This treatment puts all your affected furniture into a big, zip up bag, which is then filled with extremely hot air. This will kill the mites and their eggs. You can talk to Service Master about this, or look online at sites like Allergy Matters. See the back of this book for a list of useful contacts.

Putting things in the tumble drier is also effective, as scientists have shown that hot air can kill mites just as well as hot water. Keep something tumbling for ten minutes on hot and you should have killed off the mites.

Damp and mould

Dehumidifiers are good, but you can also try getting rid of houseplants, as the damp, mouldy spores from the earth can be damaging to sensitive lungs. Alternatively, choose leafy (not polleny) plants and cover the earth in small stones to keep the spores in the pot. Christmas trees think it's spring when they're brought into your home, and release spores that may cause asthma symptoms.

Avoid drying washing on radiators. Don't trap the warm, damp air you exhale in the house – you need to have a circulation of fresh, dry air. Any mould patches on the walls or ceiling will need to be dealt with as a priority. Get rid of fruit and veg that is decomposing in the fruit basket or fridge, air your bedding, watch out for the damp and mould that lurks in bathroom corners and at the bottom of shower curtains. Also, try not to leave damp towels hanging about.

Washing

Wash bedding at high temperatures, at least 60 degrees. (It might be an idea to change to a washing ball or natural powders for those with allergies.) Clothes that are in contact with allergens like those in cat hair need to be washed. Try not to let the kids hang around the house in their pyjamas – you are trying to keep their bedroom and bed allergen free. If you can, put the washing machine, clothes horse or tumble dryer into an outhouse or garage - it will be much better for the environment in the house. If you can 'outsource' your washing, great.

Heating

I was going to advise limiting the heating, as it promotes humidity and also makes you less inclined to let heat out by opening the windows. BUT scientists have found that if you heat your home to 72°, making mites very active, and at the same time lower your humidity below 50 per cent relative humidity (with a dehumidifier), the active mite will stay active, dry out and die of dehydration. Just the same as someone walking in the desert sun. Sounds a bit complicated though – make a judgement according to your lifestyle!

Beds and bedding

Beds need to have an airflow around them, so try not to shove them right against the wall. Wooden framed or slatted beds are healthier than divans, and mites cannot thrive in an air or water mattress.

Normal mattresses can be covered in micro porous covers, which don't allow house dust mite allergens to make contact with you. You can buy these at reasonable prices in big supermarkets, chemists and most department stores.

Pillows can be foam or feather, although it has been shown that mites colonise foam pillows more quickly. It's thought that this may be due to the much tighter weave of material encasing the feathers. Either way, wash or freeze them regularly, and cover them with micro porous slips. Ideally, you should replace them every few months.

Duvets need similar treatment, although you will probably replace them less often, so keep them covered with micro porous covers, free of pet allergens, regularly washed (probably at the laundrette) and hang them out on sunny days.

Each day, air the bed to reduce humidity and dark hiding places for mites. Simply don't make the bed – turn back the covers and let some air and sunshine in there.

You can now buy pillows and bedding with anti mite chemicals in them, and this is something you can only decide about according to your own preferences and allergies.

Linen baskets

If you're anything like me, there tends to be a constant layer of washing at the bottom of your linen basket. Unfortunately for wash-day haters, this is an ideal breeding ground for dust mites as it is damp, dark and has loads of your mouldy skin cells in it to eat! Some linen baskets are of the type that can be washed. Try to vacuum or wash underneath them regularly and not have dirty washing hanging around too long.

Pets

Pets can be a big health hazard living in our modern, un-aired environment. No pets in bedrooms, or on the sofa please! Their fur sticks to clothes and follows you around all day. You need to wash your hands and face after contact. It would definitely be healthier if they slept outside rather than in the house. Groom them regularly (outside, preferably with a damp cloth) to keep the allergens in the house at a minimum. People with allergies will usually benefit hugely if the cat, dog or other furry or feathered friends go to live somewhere else. It will take a real load off the housework, too.

Dusting and cleaning

If it's possible, change your vacuum cleaner to one with a good micro porous filter that does not send dust back out into the room. A non-asthmatic person should do the cleaning, or wear a mask or scarf if they are the only person able to do it. Don't re-use bags.

Dusting will be more effective if you do it before vacuuming. If you use a traditional dusting cloth, put it through the wash after each dusting.

While you're cleaning, using sprays or decorating, it is always advisable to have windows open. You are stirring allergens up and adding chemicals to the atmosphere, so you need to get them out of the house, not resettled somewhere else.

Think about the kind of polish and cleaning products you use, not just in the house, but for yourself. Avoid things that are stuffed with perfumes and chemicals. Again, see the back of the book for natural cleaning products.

Take action!

1. Identify which of the above points is relevant to you and your home.

2. Prioritise – which do you think is the most important thing to get sorted out, and which is least important?

3. Make a blitz list.

---

4. And start NOW – before your brain gets bunged up with other stuff. This is very important for your health, now and in the future. How hard can it be?

Giving yourself rewards for tasks completed will help!

Outside The Home
Work

At work, make sure that your working environment is well aired, especially if you are surrounded by printing, copying or computer equipment, which can produce a lot of heat and high ozone levels.

Gadget alert – there's now something called 'Nozone' which neutralises ozone. It looks like an air freshener and might help you in the office and the car. See housdustmite.org.

If possible you should ask to sit near a sunny window and have it open. If the office is air conditioned, this should keep the place reasonably dry and allergen free – although colds seem to go round and round in air conditioned places, so I would say fresh air is better, where possible.

Plants in the office should have small stones or beads over the top of the soil, to prevent mould spores flying about in the atmosphere. If that's taken care of, leafy plants are a healthy addition to office space.

Try not to keep masses of dusty papers and files around, as this is a haven for damp or storage mite. If it's necessary to keep work papers at hand, ask if you can them stored in a place away from your desk.

If you're a baker, farmer, or someone who works in fumes or with chemicals, please think very carefully about the health effects of your work and how to limit them. There's no point in being gung-ho – if you're suffering from allergies caused by your work, you need to take action. Give your immune system a break. Masks may help, or improving product storage conditions and ventilation. Consider your health versus your career.

Just don't go there!

There are obviously some places an asthmatic person just can't spend any time in. My parents' house is a case in point; it's an old, dusty farmhouse with cats and dogs running around. I cannot expect my wheezy mother in law to ever spend any time there. See, it's not always negative! Similarly, most old pubs are smoky and have small windows, open fires, a dog.. all very quaint but a definite no-no. Going there you may seem fine for a while, but will the suffering the next day be worth it?

Boring as it is, if you're an asthmatic you are going to have to stop putting your poor lungs through this kind of onslaught – have respect for the fact that there are some places you just can't be in. Go somewhere else instead, or have people around to your house. You could even be smug about everyone else poisoning themselves on cigarette smoke and breathing in the skin cells from their mangy pets. Whatever does it for you. Just stop relying on drugs to pick you up after an onslaught of allergens - do something positive to improve your health.

Young adults

It is very hard for adolescents and students to be asthmatic without being seen as a sad old party pooper by their rubbish mates. I remember insisting that my asthmatic friend came to pubs and parties with me and puffing away on fags in her presence all the while, thinking that blowing my smoke the other way was sufficient (and obviously, I was looking cool). She always had asthma attacks when she stayed over, but I never thought to keep the cats out of my bedroom in her honour. It gives me the horrors, now I know more about asthma, what effect I could have had on her health. She's gone on to be a singer, but that is definitely no thanks to my determined efforts. I wish I'd been a bit savvier at the time.

All I can suggest is that, if you have a non-asthmatic friend who keeps doing this sort of 'peer pressure' stuff to you, just tell them straight why you have to avoid these places. Explain you are trying to limit your lung damage and cut down your medication. Ask them to smoke outside when you're at the pub. Tell them their breath stinks! Whatever it takes, get people around you to be more considerate. It's also worth suggesting alternative nights out – my asthmatic friend was the only one who ever wanted to do interesting stuff that didn't involve the pub and I enjoyed her company all the more for it. Just try to avoid triggers where you can.

The Impact Of Asthma
On School Work

Asthma is a known cause of disturbed sleep, causing tiredness in the day.

Children are often the main victims of house dust mites and 'nocturnal asthma', because they spend more time in bed (where the allergens are) and because they have less capacity for understanding symptoms. They don't know that there is anything 'abnormal' about the way they feel, and they are also less able to express themselves.

Ideally, a newborn baby sleeps almost 24 hours a day and wakes only to feed. Young children of two to four years old need at least 12 hours, as well as an afternoon nap. A child between the ages of four and 12 should have between 10 to 12 hours, while a teenager of 14 to 18 years old needs about nine hours. Adults vary.

Sometimes, although a child is not wheezing or short of breath in the day, you will notice a night time cough. This can be the only manifestation of asthma, and not seem that serious – but it must be dealt with so that coughing doesn't effect daily life and progress.

These are some of the tell-tale effects of disturbed sleep that may cause psychological damage to developing children:
- Poor concentration and sleepiness
- Falling behind in schoolwork, or reducing productivity
- Moods of depression
- Restlessness
- Irritability
- Anxiety

- Heightened behavioural problems

If your kid is showing any signs of the behaviour above, it could be because he or she is over tired and feeling below par. The fact that this can result in poor schoolwork means that it can affect the child's future, so you can see how important it is to understand their health. Your actions might make a big difference to your child's performance socially, intellectually and in physical activities. In the UK, children who go to school tired and consequently fall behind in their work, have often been recommended towards 'special needs' education. This is costly, totally inappropriate and, if you take simple steps towards improving their sleep and energy levels, avoidable.

'Removing house dust mites to reduce allergic response in sensitive children may enhance their personal development and improve learning, memory, attendance, concentration and academic performance.'
(Journal of Learning Disabilities, 1993, 26 (1) p23-32)

'There is evidence that severity of asthma, persistent or severe, progresses with age. Persistent asthma at age 10 indicates persistent asthma at age 35.'
('Allergy, the Unmet Need', Royal College of Physicians' Report, June 2003)

Ensuring your kids get the right care

You should not assume that childhood asthma will be grown out of, or that it is a mere inconvenience. It needs serious thought. Simple measures to avoid allergens, and listening carefully to the doctor about how to use medication properly, should dramatically improve the quality of life for an asthmatic child.

The Global Initiative for Asthma (GINA) is doing useful work and has produced a booklet that gives doctors guidelines on how to diagnose and help families with asthmatic children. This 'Pocket Guide for Asthma Management and Prevention in Children' is a six-part asthma management programme to manage asthma in children and keep it under control. Under control means leading an active life and having proper sleep, with very few asthma attacks.

Part one of the plan deals with educating children and families about asthma care.

In **part two**, the doctor assess the seriousness of the child's asthma.

Part three of the plan involves identifying 'risk factors' – this means recognising and staying away from allergens.

Part four deals with long term medication plans.

Part five will involve setting up a personal plan to manage asthma attacks.

Part six is the regular follow up care.

You can acquire a copy of this extensive guide at www.ginaasthma.com (documents and resources section) and put your mind at rest that your doctor is providing the correct care for you and your child. If he or she is not, insist on better care or change doctors. But please remember your own part in this – some doctors are unwilling to promote allergen avoidance and will focus mainly on drugs. Please note the order of GINA's approved plan and make sure that allergen avoidance is high on **your** list of priorities. Even if you are sceptical, or your doctor is, it certainly can't hurt. In the UK there are 5.1 million people diagnosed and treated as asthmatic. 1.4 million of these are children. 80 per cent of the children are mite sensitive. Once sensitised, the house dust mite must be avoided."

Professor John Price, Asthma UK, 2002

Kids outside the home

At school, teachers should be well aware of the needs of asthmatic children. However, it is worth asking the teacher to make sure your child gets out for fresh air at break times and that his or her environment is as sunny, aired and dust free as possible. It might help you with your efforts at home if you tell the school you are changing your environment and get the teacher to keep an eye on your child's progress. It's important to ask him or her to notice how often the child uses an inhaler at school (unless the child is old enough to keep track of this). If your child is allergic to cats, try to make sure he/she is not sitting next to someone with pet cats.

Remember, the more kids that grow up knowing about the effects of allergies and pollutants, the better our asthma statistics will get.

Sleepovers at other kid's houses are a bit problematic; obviously you can't really ask to inspect the premises before you agree to the sleepover. Similarly, you can't refuse to let your child lead a normal life with friends. Maybe you could encourage friends to come to your house instead; otherwise limit the sleepovers to non-school nights for a while. Make sure that, if you or your child is going into places that are likely to be high in allergens, the correct preventor medication has been taken along and a puffer is to hand.

Chapter Six

TO HELP YOU ON YOUR WAY

Excuses, Excuses!

BUT.. It can't be my home that's the cause

- Allergic attacks come after a build up of allergens has triggered the body's defences (see Chapter Two). This means that, even if you or your family don't seem to instantly react to things like cat fur, the harmful effects of them can build up for a future 'sensitisation' leading to allergy.

- If you regularly clean your home, that's a great start. But how about the humidity of the house? Or the type of bedding you use? What you are eating? Your work or school environment? Look back at Chapter Four for advice.

- It's up to you to identify what you are allergic to. Think back to your parents house, to your office; think about your diet and read food labels.. keep a diary of what you do each day and how you feel - it helps make things clearer.

BUT.. It's too expensive to change my home around

It would be ideal to buy a dehumidifier, new mattresses, anti allergen bedding and swap your thick pile carpets for laminate flooring, amongst other things. If you can, great.. the health benefits will be worth it and you might end up spending less on medicines and childcare, etc. in the end!

However, there are plenty of basic measures you can take that don't cost much at all:

- Don't dry washing on radiators.

- Inflatable mattresses are cheap and extremely effective.
- Micro-porous covers for all bedding are really helpful.
- Open windows, air the house and lower humidity.
- Reduce hiding places for house dust mites – that means clearing clutter!
- Giving the curtains and soft furnishings a wash will be a big help.
- Most dry cleaners have carpet shampooers for hire at a reasonable cost, many with anti-allergen shampoo (check the chemicals).
- Give away your pets to good homes. Spend the money you save on pet food on a dehumidifier.

BUT.. I love Tibbles – I can't give him up

If you have pets then you probably love them and would find it terribly difficult to part with them. They are certainly not ideal living companions for anyone who suffers allergies, but if you want to keep your pets, follow these rules:

- Help your children understand why pets make them ill
- Don't let pets on the bed. No excuses.
- Don't let them into your bedroom or onto the sofas etc. Ignore 'that look' they give you – your health is far too important, isn't it?
- When the kids are ready for bed, a last minute cuddle with the cat is a big no no. Allergens from animal saliva and fur sticks to pyjamas and skin and will get directly to the bed that way. Let them say goodnight to the pets before their bath and pyjamas
- If you have a garden, the cat or dog will be fine sleeping in a kennel outside most of the year. If not, put their

bed somewhere well ventilated, preferably without carpets. The bed will need washing out regularly

- Brush or damp-wipe your pets daily to avoid their fur being spread around the house (do this outside and wash your hands afterwards)

- You might find your pets are happier for all this new attention.. but even if they give you hell, persevere! After all, with unhealthy owners, the pet's going to suffer. In fact, new evidence points to dogs and cats being victims of house dust mites and modern living conditions too. Allergies in pets, including allergic reactions to house dust mites, is rising sharply.

- Keeping caged animals indoors, including feathered friends, is definitely not recommended for people with breathing problems.

- Don't replace your pets as they pass away – getting a new puppy for Johnny is not as important as reducing his asthma.

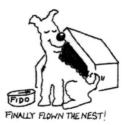

FINALLY FLOWN THE NEST!

BUT.. I'm too busy for all this extra cleaning!

It sounds daunting, especially if you are a busy working parent, to take on extra cleaning. Don't be a martyr to it;

- Explain to your family or housemates why the house needs extra cleaning

- Get the kids to do the washing up and generally take on more
- Make a rota so that everyone in the house who is able to help makes a contribution and takes the pressure off you
- Keep the rooms aired
- Don't let pets in the bedrooms or on your cushions
- Get everyone to tidy after themselves – get some boxes with lids for the clutter (which is a dust trap)
- Try to arrange it so that the asthmatic person does not do the vacuuming or dusting. (If they have to, they should wear a mask over nose and mouth to protect from dust.)

BUT.. My kids have inherited my asthma – there's nothing I can do

Don't assume that just because your asthma was not properly looked after when you were a child that things have to be the same for your family. In fact, it would be an amazing achievement to improve their health and give them chances you feel you missed out on.

- Teach them about asthma and encourage them to think about what causes it
- Think about the health benefits of the food they eat
- Keep their bedrooms and pyjamas clean and aired
- Get them away from the TV and outside to play – even if you have to bribe someone to keep an eye on them
- Outdoor games might make better presents than computer games
- Encourage them to join in activities, like swimming club, and not to feel limited by asthma

BUT.. I'm too unfit to start exercising
Or I'm scared my child will have an asthma attack if I let him/her run around

Some people only get asthma after exercise. Loads of athletes get exercise-induced asthma – possibly because of hyperventilation, bringing in great lungfulls of cold or pollen-ridden air.
But your overall health depends on keeping fit and healthy, so don't let asthma stop you exercising.

Things to remember are:

a) As a child, if you avoid things that trigger your asthma, your lung damage may be much less. This allows you to lead a normal, active life. All children should know about asthma and the allergens that commonly affect asthmatic's health – understanding why some people have breathing problems can help.
b) For unfit adults, regular, gentle exercise such as walking round the park or cycling to the shops instead of taking the car will get fresh air into your lungs and help get your general health and weight where they should be. (Avoid excessive traffic fumes). If you can do this every day you will start to build up your lung power and this will make you feel better – if you can, increase your pace, time and distance gradually. Drink plenty of water, as dehydration will make the mucous in your lungs more stringy and thick. Keep pushing yourself, gently.
c) If you are taking allergen avoidance measures and eating healthily, your symptoms, when exercising or at any other time, should decrease.
d) You can increase your muscle mass with a bit of weight lifting. Tins of beans or water bottles are a reasonable place to begin. Don't get squashed by being over enthusiastic!

e) Heart and lung function improve with exercise, asthmatic or not.

Take action!

Now you know the basics, you can make some massive changes to your health by making simple changes to your life. Don't let 'ifs' and 'buts' stop you!

Agony Aunt –
Questions From You

This is a selection of questions from the general public to Nell Nockles through our website, www.housedustmite.org, with her answers. It's interesting that some people looking for further information about house dust mites and controlling allergy are still asking about drugs. Are they after the easy way out? Tell me it isn't so!

Most of these examples are ones I have picked because they show aspects of living with allergy that you may relate to. The questions that come through also highlight the very different ways that people live! Some we get are unpleasant, but I have spared you.. just be assured that anything you can see crawling or scuttling around your house and bed is not a house dust mite.. It's something else. We get a lot of questions about this.. but house dust mites are invisible to the naked eye.

Q *Do you know what percentage of common house dust is actually human skin cells and flakes? I recall hearing that it was a large amount.*
A We are shedding old skin all the time. The amount found in house dust depends upon the home or office and ventilation, the amount of people living in the dwelling and what kind of flooring/furniture is in the room. The National Asthma Campaign in the UK has stated that an average adult may shed up to 1.5 grams of skin in a day. This is enough to feed one million dust mites. (Asthma News April/June 2002)

Q *In researching carpet cleaning companies for office space, I came across a disturbing "fact" on a company website. Quoted from the website: "Did you know that 10% of the weight of the average pillow that you put your head on is made up of dust mites, and dead dust mite bodies, and faeces of dust mites?" I have been unable to verify this statement and I would like to know how true it is.*

A That fact is from a study on old pillows (five years old) Dr Jill Warner spoke about it on a television programme in the UK. Pillows infested with mites and their debris can be a problem. Best to start out with a new pillow, cover it with micro porous material and hot wash the cover regularly. A trip to the freezer for the pillow is a good idea too.

Q *My husband has been diagnosed with a dust mite allergy and has had several reactions over the past 6 years. We have taken all the household precautions to reduce the dust mite population in our home (we live in Maryland). His allergist has suggested relocating to a state with a drier climate. Would this prove beneficial for his condition?*
A Have you considered his office as a potential source of the exacerbation of his allergy?

Q *There are so many different products to use for vacuuming etc. How is a consumer to know what is the best cleaner to use?*
A Look for awards in quality controls. In the UK there is the British Allergy Foundation that will recommend products of merit. Wherever you are located, there must be a register of products that have met stringent tests. No matter what product you use to vacuum dust particles, please remember to do this activity with a window or door open. The draft that this creates will help disperse disturbed particles away from sensitive people and outside where they cannot cause harm.

NB The British Allergy Foundation has a very helpful website with product recommendations, and we have now selected some products to sell at housedustmite.org.

Q *Doctors haven't been able to help in the slightest and all the other herbal and pill-based products that I have been dumb enough to buy have also failed. I do live in a very dusty house, with a very old carpet and everything...I am moving out for University dorms in a few months, maybe that might be the trick, of my body just being too stuffed with dust mites* *where I current live, but surely there are powerful antihistamine drugs that can lessen the symptoms and therefore reduce the shadows aren't there? I'm at the middle of discussing to buy a medication like that called "Zyrtec". Its website is www.zyrtec.com. Its one of my only hopes...*

A Sorry, it is beyond the scope of this site to recommend medication. However, it is good to hear that you are going to change your environment soon. That is one BIG step in the right direction. All the best.. ps Don't sleep with mites!

NB This guy says that NOTHING else has worked. It's hardly surprising, since he's immersing himself in his own personal poison day after day. Allergen avoidance is essential to anyone hoping to improve their allergic reactions.

Q *I have recently been told that a rash I've had for fifteen years is caused by dust mites. Is this possible? Is there any help for the itching which is unbearable.*

A Doctors say, "it is not the sore that causes the itch but itch that causes the sore". This is an allergic reaction caused by something in the environment or something that your have eaten. Most allergic people are allergic to several things. Do you know exactly what you are allergic too? It may be more than just mites you need to avoid. As far as relief from the itch, you'll have to visit your doctor for that advice. He/she should help. Please eat plenty of fruit and veg. This will help (that is, if your not allergic to these!

Q *I'm allergic to dust and have asthma. Can dust also contribute to or cause other problems that I have like eczema and arthritis? I really want to find the cause of these other two problems but so far modern medicine has been little help. If I know what the cause is I can avoid it. All my allergist wants to do is prescribe drugs rather than help me find the causes. Any suggestions? Thank you.*

A Recommend that you seek an alternative allergist who is willing to do testing for the triggers of your allergy then offer you a treatment based upon that knowledge.

Q *Can severe aches in all my body be caused by house dust etc?? The reason that I suspect this is that three different occasions of sleeping in rooms that had not been opened up to air, or been cleaned for some time, I suffered from aches & pains so bad I had a hard time to get out of bed. When going outside in fresh air I started to feel much better in a few hours. I have not seen this symptom listed anywhere so this is why I'm asking this question. My mother lives in a house that closed up all winter. She is suffering so much from aches & pains that she can hardly get out of bed. I think a good house cleaning would help, but she says no. I have slept in her bedroom & experienced the same symptoms until I gave the room a very good cleaning. She might feel better it I could clean the room. If you agree that this might help her feel somewhat better she might let me clean it !!*

A Please go to your doctor and ask for an allergy test to house dust mites and mould. Good ventilation in living space is always recommended highly by doctors. Have your mother talk to an allergist/doctor to confirm this.

Q *I have heard that a dead dust mite releases toxins. If I dry my bed sheets in the sun, which, if I understand correctly from the information you provide, will kill the dust mite, will the dead dust mite just stay on the bed sheet and merrily release toxins? Also, will sun-drying kill its eggs. What happens to its faeces with sun-drying?*

A The body parts of the mite can be allergenic but not as potent as the droppings. A good hot wash will destroy mites, eggs and wash away body parts and droppings. Please remember, it is easy to reduce mite colonies once you understand how they live. The house dust mite is 80% water. Man has lived with the mite for a very long time, it is a scavenger and to try to get rid of every one would be nearly impossible........ To concentrate on reducing potential nesting sites is advised. The mite's droppings are water-soluble. Without water, they'll usually stay intact, like a very tiny baseball, loaded with enzymes and bits.

Q *I was just diagnosed today as being allergic to dust mites. My symptoms, however, are not the usual symptoms of sneezing and coughing - my nose and my cheeks swell. Because I have been on nasal decongestants and antihistamines, the allergist said the only direction I have to go is weekly allergy shots to build up my immunity. Is that the only thing I can do, or are there other options?*

A It is important for you to reduce your exposure to house dust mites. Please read the site thoroughly and take the practical advice on offer. It may be in your interest to get another opinion on your allergy and how to treat it from another doctor. Taking 'shots' for allergy is an area of treatment that is still in debate, especially if you are allergic to more than one substance.

Q *I am allergic to house mites at a moderate level. I am wondering if they can cause a rash that comes and goes?*

A With a rash that comes and goes you are probably reacting to something else as well as mites, perhaps in your diet. The best advice is to know your allergies (visit your doctor to find out what they are) ...and avoid them. Please remember that the rash may be the result of something you had contact with hours ago...so detective work is required! Good luck!

Chapter Seven

FOR FURTHER RESEARCH

A-Z of Natural Healers

A key factor in addressing the use of supplements, choosing treatments or changing your diet will probably be total confusion. Because funded research focuses on drug therapies, there is little absolute, doctor-approved evidence that something like eating more oranges definitely reduces asthma symptoms.

Most of the foods, lifestyle changes and dietary supplements that are said to have a good (or bad) effect on asthma symptoms have been tested in small, independent studies. These are not regarded as 'conclusive', although, as could be seen in the Pilgrim Bed study, results often speak for themselves. You can choose whether to regard or disregard them.

Most of the activities, foods and supplements that are said to be good for asthmatics are those that should be part of a healthy lifestyle for everyone. Through medication, modern living, changes in fashionable foods and other factors, we are often missing out on nutrients and 'down time' that we need for optimal health.

This list will hopefully encourage you to think more carefully about eating five to eight portions of fruit or vegetable each day – it's not just a weight thing. If you want to research supplements please consult you doctor before launching into the unknown. This is just a taster – there is masses of information around, so go find it. But remember, the key is to actually start thinking about what you are doing to your body.

A

Vitamin A is one of the antioxidants we need to help protect against free radical damage, to which allergy sufferers are particularly susceptible. Also known as retinol, it is of huge importance to our skin and eyes, but asthmatics should be especially aware of it. It keeps the protective epithelial cells in the lungs intact. Low levels of vitamin A are thought to play a part in the wrong shift from TH1 to TH2 response, which is responsible for the over reaction of the immune system.

B1

B1, or Thiamin is necessary for you to effectively process fat, carbohydrates and proteins, keeping your metabolism healthy. It's in pulses, fish and meat and B complex supplements.

B6

Vitamin B6 (pyridoxine) deficiency has shown up in asthmatics. This could be because asthma drugs theophylline and aminophylline may deplete B6. A supplement has been shown to reduce asthma symptoms. It's in turkey, tuna, potatoes, liver, lentils and bananas.

B12

Vitamin B12 can help those who have a reaction to sulphates (food and drink additives) which may be making asthma symptoms worse. Meat, fish and dairy will help you get your B12 levels right.

Boswellia

A small study has indicated that asthma and breathing capacity can be improved by taking this herb, as it has anti-flammatory properties and inhibits leukotrines.

Buyteko

The famous Russian Buyteko Breathing Technique is designed to correct the oxygen and carbon dioxide imbalance in asthma. Dr Buyteko believes that too much oxygen, from poor breathing habits, causes many symptoms of asthma. His technique corrects the imbalance. Buyteko breathing techniques have improved the lives of many asthmatics, and it is claimed a few have been completely cured. It has been more extensively tested than most other non medical methods. There are numerous books about it, and it is usually recommended that asthmatics (or anyone suffering breathing difficulty) should go on an approved course to learn these shallow breathing techniques.

C

Vitamin C is an antioxidant and anti inflammatory which can influence the development of asthma symptoms. In preliminary studies, children eating a diet rich in fruits and vegetable with high vitamin C content have had significantly less wheezing. It might work better for some asthma sufferers in the form of sodium ascorbate or calcium ascorbate rather than its usual form, ascorbic acid.

Calcium

Calcium levels must be maintained if you take corticosteroids, as one of their possible side effects is osteoporosis. Fish (especially sardines), vegetables and milk are calcium-rich foods. Ask for advice about supplements if you prefer.

Camomile extract

A soothing anti-inflammatory.

E

Vitamin E is a major antioxidant, helping to prevent every part of you from free radical damage. It's extremely effective, especially when it's backed up by selenium, vitamin c and beta-carotene. It inhibits leukotrienes and blocks the activation of some of the inflammatory cells that produce them. Wholegrain cereals, eggs, leafy greens, egg yolks, nuts and seeds are all good sources. It's widely available as a supplement.

Eucalyptus oil

A few drops in with the washing powder helps to kill house dust mites in all your machine washable items.

Fish oil

Great news for kids everywhere.. a dose of cod liver oil each day is a good idea, because it's an anti-inflammatory. Because of the massive proven benefit to brain function, fish oil supplements are now available in various tasteless or even citrussy forms. Become a non-wheezy brainiac!Get to the chemist or health food shop..Or the fishmonger.. mackerel, tuna, trout or salmon are ideal oily fish, full of Omega 3 fatty acids, and the wild (non-farmed) ones are best. It's been suggested that asthma levels in Japanese are low because they eat lots of sushi (raw fish). A study published in the Medical Journal of Australia in 1996 found that children who ate oily fish once a week had a 75 per cent reduced risk of asthma symptoms.

Flavanoids

Antioxidants from plants that help us to absorb vitamin C. See 'Green'.

Gingko biloba

Can help open bronchial tubes and let you breathe more easily. It blocks the platelet activating factor that adds to asthma symptoms. GB is credited with getting blood circulating properly, particularly for the extremities and the brain.

Grape seed

Extract of grape seed contains caffeine and theophylline, both of which may help to relieve bronchial tightening.

Green

I include all green vegetables in 'green'. They contain alpha and beta carotene, lutien and zeaxanthin, flavanoids, querticin, vitamins A, C and E. Fussy kids can be easily fooled into eating veg if you liquidise it up with tomatoes (spaghetti Bolognese, soups etc). Sounds horrible, tastes nice. Don't overcook the veg and try to use the 'green water' for making gravy and sauce instead of throwing it away. Kids also tend to be quite fond of crudités - cut-up sticks of raw veg.

Green lipped mussel

The new black, apparently this is the extract of choice for celebrity asthmatics. It is suggested that the glycosaminoglycans in the mussels, which are only found in New Zealand (told you it was posh), can maintain and rebuild connective tissues and have anti inflammatory properties. Apart from it helping asthma, people are also having good results in treating arthritis and injury recovery. Warning: shellfish allergy could make this one a bad idea; you **must** get your allergies tested and get advised on taking this.

Lobelia

One of the oldest asthma and cough treatments, lobelia is used as an anti spasmodic.

Magnesium

Proven to be a massive benefit to asthmatics, it helps calm down tightness and prevent spasm in the bronchial passages. It may also stabilise the mast cells and T lymphocytes in your angry immune system. It's found in beans, dairy, meat, nuts, cereals and green veg.

Onion

An anti-inflammatory, with quercetin.

Quercetin

Quercitin is a flavanoid contained in most plants. It inhibits leukotrienes and blocks histamine release – both of these are trouble makers in the allergic response. It's in supplements, or naturally found in apples, tea, onions, vegetables and pulses.

Rosemary

Reduces muscle constriction in the throat and airways.

Thymus

The Thymus gland is in your neck, so it knows a thing or two about the immune system. It regulates the cells that go crazy when they sense invasion. Speak to the doctor about this one.

Saiboku-to

This old Japanese herbal formula has been found to reduce asthma symptoms and can help people reduce their use of steroids, because of its anti-inflammatory properties. It would be worth talking to a Chinese or Japanese herbalist about such asthma remedies and making your own informed judgements about them.

Salt

No, stop! This must be regulated, as you know, and it's especially important for men to watch out, as they have been found more susceptible to the increase in airway reactivity that can come about from too much salt. Watch out for high sodium levels, particularly in ready meals and shop-bought soups and sandwiches. Kids love salty, sugary food, so if you have a small one, try to wean him or her off early before you go too far down the spaghetti hoop road.

Selenium

A couple of brazil nuts a day could be all you need to keep your selenium levels optimal, or get the supplement if you're allergic to nuts. This important trace mineral protects against free radical damage and is very powerful alongside its old pal vitamin E.

Spirulina
Spirulina is a good source of flavanoids with the anti-inflammatory and antioxidant effects that could benefit asthmatics.

Tomatoes
Stuffed with antioxidants, beta-carotene, which prevents free radical damage, and lycopene, which can help reduce asthma symptoms brought on by exercise.

Yoga
Yoga involves stretching and some weight bearing. It focuses on bodily strength and control and good breathing techniques. It also helps 'calm your nerves' – thought to be a trigger for some. You can do it at home (get a book or video) and it's not just for girls.

Zinc
Zinc is a healer – it can shorten the duration of a common cold, as well as boost the immune system and act as an antioxidant.

GOOD LUCK!

BOOKS

'Asthma: Relax – You're Not Going To Die'
Jonathan M Berkowitz, MD
ISBN 1591200237

'House Dust Mites - How they affect asthma, eczema and other allergies'
Des Whitrow
ISBN 0716020343

'The Complete Guide To Asthma'
Jonathan Brostoff, Linda Gamlin
ISBN 074754438

'Freedom from Asthma: Buteyko's Revolutionary Treatment'
Alexander Stalmatski, Kyle Cathie, Foreword by Konstantin Buteyko
ISBN 1856263355

'My House is Killing Me! – The home guide for families with allergy and asthma'
Jonathan Samet (Foreword), Jeffrey C May
ISBN 0801867290

'Prescription for Nutritional Healing – A practical A-Z reference to drug free remedies using vitamins, herbs and food supplements'
Phyllis Balch, James F Balch
ISBN 1583330771

USEFUL INFORMATION

www.housedustmite.org	**House dust mites & asthma**
www.GINA.org	**Global Initiative for Asthma**
www.lung.ca/asthma	**The Lung Association (Canada)**
www.environmental-assistance.org	**Damp, indoor and outdoor environment**
www.asthma.org	**Asthma UK (National Asthma Campaign)**
www.eczema.org	**The National Eczema Society**
www.talkeczema.com	**Talk Eczema**
www.eczema.org.au	**Exzema Association of Australia**
www.allergyfoundation.com	**Allergy UK (British Allergy Foundation)**
www.insectresearch.com	**Insect R & D Ltd**
www.bad.org.uk	**British Association of Dermatologists**
www.1stvitality.co.uk	**Non-drug advice**

www.aaaai.org

American Academy of Allergy, Asthma and Immunology

PRODUCTS & SERVICES

www.housedustmite.org	**Products**
www.ebac.com	**Dehumidifiers**
www.healthyflooring.net	**The Carpet Foundation**
www.sbsoftwaresystems.com	**'Asthmalyser' software**
www.allergymatters.co.uk	**All types of allergies, information & safe products**
www.healthguardtm.co.uk	**Spray for furniture and beds**
www.servicemaster.co.uk	**Anti-allergen heat treatment**
www.allergybegone.com	**Various products**
www.lyprinol.co.uk	**Product (green lipped mussel extract)**
www.nutrient.co.uk	**Nutrients**
www.airpurifiers.co.uk	**Products and general allergen information**
www.aquaball.com	**Natural washing and cleaning products**
www.healthy-house.co.uk	**Natural domestic and anti- allergen products**
www.atmospherics.co.uk	**'Nozone' – to eliminate ozone in confined**

spaces

www.babygaia.co.uk	**Mother and baby friendly products**
www.ecopaints.com	**allergy friendly paints**
www.medicalert.org.uk	**UK help service and ID bracelets in case of emergency**

www.medicalert.org   **USA help service and
                            ID bracelets in case of
                            emergency**

www.theipcrg.org   **International Primary
                            Care Respiritory Group**

                       –

                            **Lots of links for lots of
                            countries**

HELPLINES

Asthma UK Helpline (for all asthma-related advice) 0845 7010203

NHS Direct (for fast medical advice) 0845 46 47

British Allergy Foundation (all allergy advice) 020 8303 8583

SAMPLE ALLERGY DIARY

Filling in something simple along these lines will help you keep track and get in control.

Week commencing / / Monday		
Peak Flow am	Reading:	Percent of best:
Activities		
Places & people		
Food & drink		
Medication taken		
Peak Flow pm	Reading:	Percent of best:
How you feel:		
How you slept:		
Why your symptoms are good/bad:		
What you found out:		
Tuesday		
Peak Flow am	Reading:	Percent of best;
Activities		
Places & pople		
Food & drink		
Medication taken		
Peak Flow pm	Reading:	Percent of best::
How you feel:		
How you slept:		
Why your symptoms are good/bad:		
What you found out:		

Wednesday		
Peak Flow am	Reading:	Percent of best::
Activities		
Places & people		
Food & drink		
Medication taken		
Peak Flow pm	Reading:	Percent of best::
How you feel: How you slept: Why your symptoms are good/bad: What you found out:		

Thursday		
Peak Flow am	Reading:	Percent of best::
Activities		
Places & people		
Food & drink		
Medication taken		
Peak Flow pm	Reading:	Percent of best::
How you feel: How you slept: Why your symptoms are good/bad: What you found out:		

Friday		
Peak Flow am	Reading:	Percent of best::
Activities		
Places & people		

Food & drink		
Medication taken		
Peak Flow pm	Reading:	Percent of best::

How you feel:

How you slept:

Why your symptoms are good/bad:

What you found out:

Saturday

Peak Flow am	Reading:	Percent of best::
Activities		
Places & people		
Food & drink		
Medication taken		
Peak Flow pm	Reading:	Percent of best::

How you feel:

How you slept:

Why your symptoms are good/bad:

What you found out:

Sunday

Peak Flow am	Reading:	Percent of best::
Activities		
Places & people		
Food & drink		
Medication taken		
Peak Flow pm	Reading:	Percent of best::

How you feel:
How you slept:
Why your symptoms are good/bad:

What you found out:

REFERENCES

Full referencing and research notes are available by enquiry, or visit the research areas of housedustmite.org.

As always, those who wish to research supplements or alternative therapies should seek specialised information on those subjects according to their own personal circumstances.

Useful books and websites are listed on the previous page. Please make contact with us via housedustmite.org, or rosie@nockles.com, with specific questions.